GERONTOLOGY

and the

CONSTRUCTION

of OLD

AGE

GERONTOLOGY
and the
CONSTRUCTION
of OLD
AGE

With a new introduction
by Roberta R. Greene
and Robert G. Blundo

BRYAN S. GREEN

ALDINET**RANSACTION**
A Division of Transaction Publishers
New Brunswick (U.S.A.) and London (U.K.)

Library of Congress Catalog Number: 2009015499
ISBN: 978-0-202-36255-7
Printed in the United States of America

Library of Congress Cataloging-in-Publication Data

Green, Bryan S. R.
    Gerontology and the construction of old age / Bryan S. Green ; with a new introduction by Roberta R. Greene and Robert G. Blundo.
        p. cm.
    Includes bibliographical references and index.
    ISBN 978-0-202-36255-7 (acid-free paper)
        1. Gerontology. 2. Discourse analysis. I. Title.

HQ1061.G714 2009
305.26–dc22

                                                            2009015499

To my grandmother, Elizabeth Millard

Contents

3   THE GRAMMAR OF DEPENDENCE AND CARE
    IN GERONTOLOGY

4   MECHANISMS OF FIELD ORGANIZATION
    IN GERONTOLOGY

5   DISPERSAL AND INTEGRATION OF "THE AGED"
    IN GERONTOLOGICAL DISCOURSE

Introduction to the Transaction Edition

We have arranged for ourselves a world in which we can live—by positing bodies, lines, planes, causes and effects, motion and rest, form and content; without the articles of faith nobody now could endure life. But that does not prove them. Life is no argument. The conditions of life might include errors.

—Friedrich Nietzsche (1974, p. 177)

In the welcome second edition of his text *Gerontology and the Construction of Old Age*, Bryan Green adroitly employs the lens of constitutive realism as a tool to analyze professional discourse, providing a background for the reader to examine the language of gerontology. Green challenges the philosophy of modernity and Cartesian certainty that knowledge lies outside of ourselves and only needs to be discovered. He counters this with Foucault's (1970, 1976) postmodern view that knowledge is constructed through day-to-day discourse—speaking, hearing, writing, and reading. In keeping with this idea, Green contends that all social science, in this case gerontology, is created by the very language it speaks. For those gerontologists who have not considered the ideas of constitutive realism, this book introduces many new thoughts about how language can shape the very identity of the profession.

As a postmodern thinker, Green takes the perspective that "reality" cannot exist independent of the complexity of peoples' narratives within a given culture. Cultural bias, values, myth, metaphor, power, and political context all come into play as people go about the day's business, although these people may believe and act as if they are seeing and experiencing an actual independent reality (Blundo & Greene, 2008). That is, postmodernists believe that what we know, our fundamental knowledge, is created at the level of ongoing narratives, unlike positivists, who argue for universal truths and assume that values, beliefs, and sociopolitical issues exist independent of language and constructive dialogical processes.

Discourse, as discussed by Green, refers to a systematic way of providing parameters for what can be known, said, and thought of at a particular historical moment (Chambon, Irving, & Epstein, 1999). The focus is on "how social reality is achieved, produced, or constructed, and by what means" a profession is constituted (Green, 1993, p. 14). That is, Green examines how gerontologists create their profession, taking momentary and contextual ideas about "the aged" and fashioning a social reality named *gerontology*.

In other words, Green uses language as the unit of analysis to be explored or as an organizing phenomenon in its own right. In short, he examines gerontology"as a field of discourse embodied in texts and realized in reading effects"(Green, 1993, p. 9).The very research, theories, and literature produced within gerontology and viewed as knowledge within the field are, in fact, what we label gerontology.

Green's analysis provides the reader with profound and disturbing ideas about how gerontologists use language. For example, the use of the definite article *the* before the word *aged* takes on a complex meaning. Green declares that"the aged"is a master category. By *master category*, he means a form of linguistic shorthand, a heuristic that"bound(s), organize(s), authorize(s) and collect(s) topics into a single framework"(Greene, 1993, p. 151). By"naming" older adults as"the aged,"the author assures the reader that there is a field of study focused on a linguistically constructed concept of human beings. The use of this master category provides the focal point for a group of people who maintain a field of study named gerontology. In this way, master categories engage the reader with a familiar construct.

For example, Green calls our attention to a chapter title in a handbook on "the ageing."He notes that the diverse areas of interest and practice included in the chapter, such as housing, health, economics, and so on, are held to-gether by this master category. The master category also brings unity to the profession and a range of areas of interest to those who consider themselves gerontologists. Green (1993) notes that"what becomes incredible for geron-tology is the capacity for a single term, the aged, to conceptually embrace so many services and facilities as those now provided or to provide an adequate common denominator of them all"(p. 135).

The naming of the discipline gerontology and its related texts and concepts as well as the setting of common points of reference and boundaries, such as what constitutes aging and old age in its many permutations over the years, give legitimacy to the field. Ordinary language is"inscribed"upon or rewritten in the language of the profession. Green makes the argument that gerontology was designated a legitimate field of inquiry partly when growing old and being older became more commonplace in modern society. Ordinary language no longer sufficed to make the phenomenon comprehensible.That is,"social science shows itself to be a higher order of knowledge by conspicu-ously transcending the mundane level of what every member pragmatically knows"(Green, 1993, p. 33).

Green uses constitutive realism to provide an example of how, despite good intentions, gerontologists may craft a language that denigrates older adults. A discussion of the"care-dependency continuum"provides readers with penetrating new insights into how gerontologists have engaged in the creation of the idea that"the aged"are people who need someone to care for them.Those older adults who refuse service from altruistic service providers are"resistant."These predetermined"needs"of"the elderly"are in turn a sign of"dependency."

Bryan Green contends that negative images of older adults permeate the array of public programs known as the *aging enterprise* (Estes, 1979). One must agree with Green that in societies that value youth and individual responsibility rather than stress collective responsibility, government entitlements take on a different character. In an individualistic society, such as the United States, discourse is, as Green (1993) says, "around the care-dependency circuit" (p. 103). In collective societies, such as Sweden, the political language of "home," "shelter," and "security" prevails.

Moreover, Green challenges us when he argues that there is an implicit agreement among gerontologists about old-age policy. This familiar "contract" puts forth the idea that care exists on a measurable continuum running from independence to dependence. Not only is care measurable, it is a distributable entity subject to the language of supply and demand, cost-benefit analysis, and rationale delivery systems. This raises an important question: Are we locked in policy debates that Bryan Green says renders older adults frail and dependent, or can older adults expect us to understand their expressed wants?

Green is describing a conundrum with which any profession, in this case gerontology, must contend if and only if it wishes to ask "What is this we do?" He does say that language lends itself to rational mastery and control and that we can question the precepts of the profession and our policy constructs if we work for our professional ideals. Calling attention to our negative portrayal of older adults is not new. Robert Butler (1975), a psychiatrist and the first director of the National Institute on Aging, is perhaps the most well-known combatant of the negative stereotyping of older adults. He believed that this negativity was so pervasive, particularly among professionals, that he coined the term *ageism* to address this prejudice. In another discussion related to ageism among professional social workers, Greene (2008) also cautioned that the therapeutic relationship could be jeopardized when irrational images of older adults disrupt the communication process. In addition, postmodern-oriented family therapists have warned that negative societal attitudes such as ageism can distort the therapeutic conversation.

In the 1950s, as the field of gerontology expanded and became multidisciplinary, the process of scientific inquiry required language that embodied institutional categories, a distinct nomenclature, and descriptive protocols. Diagnoses and prognoses were thought to be part of the formation of human sciences. Thus, gerontology became a new area of scientific inquiry, with scientists defining aging as a disease, seemingly lodging gerontology in a scientific clinical vocabulary.

Until the late 1980s, gerontology was dominated by the perspective that growing old is a time of decline and loss. But during the 1970s and 1980s, the view that equated aging with disease began to be countered with a more hopeful philosophy. In 1987 the publication of Rowe and Kahn's *Successful Aging* added loud voice to the idea that aging is not a "disease." The notion was put forth that if individuals adopted healthy behaviors, they could advance to old age with far fewer age-associated diseases (Strawbridge, Wallhagen, & Cohen, 2002). Crowther, Parker, Achenbaum, Larimore, and Koenig (2002) further proposed that maximizing positive spirituality could contribute to successful aging.

During more recent decades, gerontologists have made significant strides in advancing a wellness philosophy. Antonovsky (1998) used the phrase *salu-togenesis orientation* to characterize his study of how people can naturally use their internal resources to strive for health. Similarly, Atchley (1999) proposed the idea of life continuity, in which older adults maintain their thinking patterns, activities, living arrangements, and social relationships despite changes in health. Yet one might agree with Bryan Green that the efforts to advance a positive image of aging have left us with mixed images of aging, with the language of gerontology exposing a chronic ambivalence about older adults.

This revision of Green's text provides an opportunity for those in the field of gerontology to look at a timeless deconstruction of gerontology with all its implications for research, practice, and policy if only the field has the courage to look seriously into its own foundations of thought and practice. This is not an easy task for any profession to undertake, for it challenges many values and ideas upon which the practitioner and the field base their practice. We hope that this new printing will give the practitioners of gerontology an opportunity to take a hard look at what the field might look like given these insights.

Roberta R. Greene
Robert G. Blundo

References

Antonovsky, A. (1998). The sense of coherence: An historical and future perspective. In H. I. McCubbin, E. A. Thompson, A. I. Thompson, & J. E. Fromer (Eds.), *Stress, Coping, and Health in Families* (pp. 3–20). Boston: Allyn & Bacon.

Atchley, R. C. (1999). *Continuity and Adaptation in Aging: Creating Positive Experiences.* Baltimore: Johns Hopkins University Press.

Blundo, R., & Greene, R. R. (2008). Social construction. In R. R. Greene (Ed.), *Human Behavior Theory and Social Work Practice* (3rd ed., pp. 237–264). New Brunswick, NJ: Aldine Transaction.

Butler, R. N. (1975). *Why Survive? Being Old in America.* New York: Harper & Row.

Chambon, A. S., Irving, A., & Epstein, L. (1999). *Reading Foucault for Social Work.* New York: Columbia University Press.

Crowther, M. R., Parker, M. W., Achenbaum, W. A., Larimore, W. L., & Koenig, H. G. (2002). Rowe and Kahn's model of successful aging revisited: Positive spirituality–The forgotten factor. *The Gerontologist*, 42, 613–620.

Estes, C. (1979). *The Aging Enterprise.* San Francisco: Jossey Bass.

Foucault, M. (1970). *The Order of Things: An Archaeology of the Human Sciences* (Alan Sheridan, Trans.). New York: Pantheon.

Foucault, M. (1976). *Mental Illness and Psychology* (Alan Sheridan, Trans.). New York: Harper & Row.

Green, B. S. (1993). *Gerontology and the Construction of Old Age: A Study in Discourse Analysis* (1st ed.). New York: Walter de Gruyter.

Greene, R. R. (2008). *Social Work with the Aged and Their Families. 3rd edition* New Brunswick, NJ: Aldine Transaction.

Nietzsche, F. (1974). *The Gray Science.* Translated by Walter Kaufman. New York: Vintage.

Rowe, J. W., & Kahn, R. L. (1987). Successful aging. *Science,* July, 237 (4811), 143-149.

Strawbridge, W. J., Wallhagen, M. I., & Cohen, R. D. (2002). Successful aging and well-being: Self-rated compared with Rowe and Kahn. *The Gerontologist,* 42, 727–733.

Preface

This book has two aims. The first is to describe analytically an important field of study: gerontology, a phenomenon important both for its growing academic presence and for its practical effects on discourse and policy concerning old age. The second is to help develop possibilities of inquiry associated with the linguistic, literary, and rhetorical turns of social science in recent years. This will be done with specific reference to social science discourse, running parallel to comparable efforts (such as those in Brown, 1992; McClosky, 1985, 1990; Turner and Bruner, 1986; Simons, 1989, 1990), but I see the methods involved as parts of a whole strategy applicable to every topic of social inquiry, not just to the study of discourses. To this end, Chapter 1 identifies a methodological position termed constitutive realism, based on the principle that the nature of social reality is that of instanced codes, schemata, scripts and grammars—not that of substantial things.

There is, of course, nothing new about constitutive realism. The developments referred to above have turned linguistically conceived social inquiry from a relatively quiet byroad into a busy thoroughfare. This is evident in the creation of new journals such as *Discourse and Society*, *Textual Practice*, *Communication Theory*, and *Written Communication*, the increased circulation of anthologies and collections to expand the reading economy of scholars (for example, Bazerman and Paradis, 1991; Brown, 1992; Clifford and Marcus, 1986; Hunter, 1991; Law, 1986; Nelson et al., 1987; Simons, 1989, 1990; Woolgar, 1988), and the publication of special series such as that in which the present volume appears. Moreover, in view of these developments one can see, with retrospective clarity, anticipations of constitutive realism in classical sociology: in Marx's revelation of the founding categories of capitalism—especially the commodity form of value—in the discourse of political economy (for example, Marx, 1977:356–358, 415–416, 421–443), in Simmel's analysis of the "constitutive concepts of history" (Simmel, 1980:145–197) explaining how events are made into history, and his parallel analysis of how interacting subjects synthesize themselves and their actions to make social reality (Simmel, 1971:6–22), in the neo-Kantian idea that social reality is value constituted (Radbruch, 1950; Rickert, 1986), in Durkheim's theorizing of collective representations as the core of social reality (Durkheim, 1915:259–265, 305–308, 467–496; 1974:1–34), and in Durkheim's appropriation of the claim by American pragmatists, especially Dewey and James, that "we are the co-authors of reality" (Durkheim, 1983:85). Beyond classical sociology, pragmatist concepts of reality formation enter, via Mead, into symbolic interactionism and labeling theory. Also, there is Schütz's cultivation of social phenomenology (Schütz, 1967, 1973), leading into ethnomethodology, perhaps the fullest realization of constitutive realism in sociological inquiry.

The task posed, then, by constitutive realism and taken up in this study is not one of announcing a new position and persuading others to adopt it. Rather, the task is to sharpen an idea long present in sociology but displaced or clouded by the conceptual detritus of substantialist images of social reality: society as mechanism, society as organic structure, society as a cybernetic system. Ultimately, the task cannot be completed by methodological debate, however necessary this may be, but only through doing work that draws out the consequences of accepting constitutive realism. This is part of my intent and, to this end, I offer in Chapter 1 a specific version of constitutive realism.

Regarding the aim of characterizing gerontology, some caveats and disclaimers are called for so as not to be misunderstood.

First, in line with the principles of constitutive realism, I take the essential character of gerontology to lie in its determinate organization of thought in writing, in its being a formation of text and discourse, rather than in its institutional settings, organizational features, or sociopolitical applications. These are important but, for my purpose, secondary considerations. I do not, therefore, claim to offer the politics, economics, sociology, or institutional history of the field. Although centrally concerned with its concepts and theories, I adopt a configurational rather than historical perspective, being more concerned with describing its prevailing formations and how they cohere rather than how they and their components grew into existence. The latter is a complementary line of inquiry but one requiring special research and a separate study. It would require, for example, a full chronicle of texts and an identification of key writings (cf. Streib and Orbach's summary sketch, 1967), from which data base one could then write a systematic textual history and textual evolution of the field. This I have not attempted. There are allusions of this kind in Chapter 2, "The Foundations of Gerontology," but even there the term "foundations" is interpreted more in the architectural sense of currently functioning structures than of historical origins. This is reflected in the fact that although use is made there of Foucauldian ideas they are drawn from Foucault's archeology of knowledge rather than his genealogy of power/knowledge complexes. The chapter is not, therefore, Foucauldian, except in the sense of highly selective borrowing. The emphasis there, as throughout the book, is on the present structure of gerontology discourse. References to the past of the field and its context of growth are entirely subordinate to that interest.

The contrasts made in the preceding disclaimer lead to a further clarification of purpose. If the study had to be described in terms of forced choices between structural and historical, morphological and developmental, synchronic and diachronic, then the first term of each pair would have to be chosen. This would, however, make the study seem formalistic and obscure its central concern with the textual *dynamics* of gerontology and its *working* principles, the principles that set thought and communication to work in certain ways. I see gerontology discourse as an active organization of language, informed by dialectical tensions and counteractions, not as an algebraic structure of signifiers or a schematic superstructure. My interest is in the pragmatics of language use. I want to identify the compositional norms and performative compulsions of writing, reading, and doing gerontology: the semantic normalities, syntactic regularities, and linguistic constitution of the field. In Nelson Goodman's (1978) phrase, I want to identify the 'ways of worldmaking' contained in the field and binding on anyone entering it. The pragmatic interest here is that entrance to the field carries with it membership requirements of coherent utterance, rational expression, and effective communication. It is these I wish to articulate.

Nothing said above should be taken to imply that gerontologists are so insensitive to the linguistic turn or so lacking in methodological self-reflection that they need instruction from outsiders. Such advice would be impertinent and gratuitous. Practitioners of gerontology are already incorporating theories of rhetoric, discourse, metaphor, and narrative into their methodologies. For example, a collection of papers edited by Marshall (1986) includes a phenomenological model by Ryff, a Meadian perspective by Chappell and Orbach, and a symbolic interactionist approach by Spence. Contributions to the *Journal of Aging Studies* since its inception in 1987 include papers deploying rhetoric analysis (Hazan, 1988), metaphor analysis (Kraus et al., 1990), and narrative analysis (Luborsky, 1990; Manheimer, 1989; Wyatt-Brown, 1989). The 1991 Annual Conference of the Gerontological Society of America, San Francisco, California, included a symposium on 'Discourse(s) of Gerontology' with a bibliography containing references to Bazerman, Brown, Foucault, Gusfield, McClosky, Nelson, Simons, Woolgar, and others cited in the present study.

It is clear, then, that the field itself is being stirred by the linguistic turn of social science methodology. My contribution would be to reinforce such tendencies and take the turn a degree further by including the language practices through which gerontology composes a researchable subject matter and imparts objective existence to it. This is something that only an outsider can properly do. If my arguments regarding these practices and their constitutive necessity for the integrity of the field have any validity, then, as I argue in Chapter 6 with regard to critical gerontology, they will be encountered as limitations beyond which gerontology becomes inoperable. The constitutive practices will continue to assert themselves in textual performances of gerontology, regardless of programmatic dedications to radical reformation or adventurous methodological speculations. Every field of discourse has built into it principles of self-conservation as well as change, and I see textually based discourse analysis as uniquely capable of grasping them. This will be disputed by critical gerontologists or other theorists regarding discourses as first and foremost socially constructed (see, for example, Baars, 1991, and those debated in Chapter 6). For them, the principles of conservation and change will be sought outside the field of discourse, in economic structures, social hierarchies, and power relations; in the contextual structure of society rather than the internal structure of the discourse as such. Admittedly, this is a matter of strategic choice, not mutual exclusion, since one consideration will lead to the other. However, the choice whether to begin with a textual analysis and move outward or with a contextual analysis and move inward is important. My belief is that the contextual strategy is analytically dangerous precisely because of its strength. However the context is formulated (as gendered power relations, as the logic of capitalism, as interest group conflict, or something else) it will provide an interpretive frame so strong that it becomes difficult to read the texts of a field as anything but documentary indicators of contextual pattern. Reading the texts for their own structures and dynamics is thus preempted by reading them for contextual structures and dynamics already known. Their own constitutive significance for the discourse they convey is likely to be missed or even dismissed by the contextual strategy.

Having expressed a reservation about critical theory, as usually understood, and the strategy of critical gerontology, I should confess to sharing with them an intellectual conviction that is political. I believe that the greatest good of social inquiry is to serve what Habermas (1971) calls the emancipatory interest of knowledge. In particular, it can help free conduct, including the conduct of thought and language, from habitual methods and proprieties taken for granted.

The present study came to be written because I have a long-standing interest in policy reports as major means of reality and knowledge construction in modern society. Politically, they belong to the ruling apparatuses of society (see, Smith, 1990a,b) and to what Habermas (1987) calls the colonialization of the lifeworld by system rationality. In pursuing that interest, I have sought a methodological strategy for the textual analysis of policy documents, hoping in this way to induce critical reflection about them. As part of this enterprise I began, in 1988, to apply textual analysis to Canadian and American policy documents on aging and the aged. It soon became apparent, especially in the case of American reports, that they were permeated with concepts and findings from gerontology. Consequently, I began reviewing the literature as part of the linguistic environment of the reports. Once in the literature I was enthralled by its scope and richness and investigation of its texture became a project in its own right. I intend ultimately, however, to return this study to the path of policy analysis from which it departed.

Regarding the selection of texts, I cannot claim to have conducted a sample survey. I do not know of any list of the population of texts from which a sample might be drawn or what the validity of such a procedure might be. In the event, I tried to immerse myself in the literature, reading as widely as possible in currently circulating textbooks, readers, journal articles, and frequently cited works, until a sense of repetitive pattern and structural cohesion was achieved. In this sense, the procedure was something like that of an ethnographer trying to become a competent member of a language community.

* * *

Thanks are due to Judith Fraser (York University, Canada) for her assistance in exploring and charting the gerontology literature. Also, I want to acknowledge suggestions from Norbert Wiley (University of Illinois) for sharpening my version of constitutive realism and helpful criticisms from David Maines (Wayne State University), the series editor. Thanks also to Dianne Pantele at York's Secretarial Services for professionally typing the manuscript.

Introduction

To bring the object of this study into focus, I want to address the question, What is gerontology? At first it would seem sufficient to quote practitioners' definitions within the field.

> The scientific study of the biological, psychological, and social aspects of aging. Elie Metchnikroff, a biologist, coined the term in 1903 for the Greek word *geront* meaning 'old man' and 'logos' meaning 'study of.' (Harris, 1988:80)

> Gerontology is the discipline that systematically studies aging. It looks at aging from two points of view: how aging affects the individual and how an aging population will change society. (Novak, 1988:4)

The trouble with such definitions, however, is they say more about what gerontology wants to be or declares itself to be than what it is. In this sense they are glosses on the actuality of the field rather than displays of it. They leave the phenomenon of gerontology, its compositional structures, and its dynamics of discourse still to be analyzed. A starting point is given by observing that gerontology is a connected set of writings, a literature. However, since more writings are being added continually, the phenomenon cannot be equated with the literature so far. The fact that more writings can be added, that they become incorporated into a body of writings, suggests the operation of some system of literary production: methods of appropriating and articulating a subject matter, regularities of topical organization, mechanisms of field coherence, and means of field production. Since these are principles generating a literature, the methods, regularities, mechanisms, and means in question must be linguistic and textual, although not abstractly linguistic, because the literature belongs to social science and to human studies, and is thus bound to particular performative requirements of writing and reading.

Let us say then, as a guiding formulation, that gerontology is a linguistic field of discourse defined by certain practices of literary production. (I do not say this is all it is, but considerations of institutional location, professional networks, and the like belong to the social organi-

zation of the discipline not the internal constitution of the field that such
organization embodies and depends on.) Given the formulation, we
must approach the phenomenon through methods of language analysis.
At the same time it is important to preserve our sociological and political
interest in the subject matter of gerontology and in the meanings it
communicates about aging and the aged, and not succumb to a purely
scientific interest in language as such.

METHODS OF LANGUAGE ANALYSIS: AN OVERVIEW OF CONCEPTUAL RESOURCES

Given the bewildering variety of approaches to language and discourse developed in literary theory, cognitive science, semiotics, and
ethnomethodology, it will be helpful to organize an inventory of methods to take stock of the conceptual resources they offer. I will begin with
semiotics since this is the most general and inclusive approach to language analysis.

The dominant tradition in semiotics stems from Ferdinand de Saussure ([1916] 1959). Saussure claimed that semiotics (which he called
semiology) is a science of signs in general, thereby including linguistics
as a special branch dealing with verbal signs in speech and writing.
Roland Barthes (1967:9–11) argues that since every human system of
signification depends on language either as model, component or interpretive relay, semiology might better be regarded as a branch of linguistics. Either way, Saussurean linguistics is founded on the abstraction of
sign relations, values, and functions from any particular acts of use and
performance, yielding the formal kind of approach I would guard
against even though wanting to appropriate from it whatever suits the
purpose. I adopt the same predatory attitude toward scientific linguistics in general, including semiotics, that Fredric Jameson has recom-
mended toward A. J. Greimas, a French structuralist in the Saussurean
tradition whose works will be drawn on quite extensively in the present
study:

> we outsiders or interlopers—who resist the invitation to join the discipline
> and to 'become semioticians', that is, to convert to the entire Greimassian
> code . . . should also feel free to bricolate all this, that is, in plainer lan-
> guage, simply to steal the pieces that interest or fascinate us, and to carry
> off our fragmentary booty to our intellectual caves. (Jameson, 1987:viii)

Semiotics is not in principle closed off from the study of language
performance and contingent use even though this is the basis of Saus-

surean structuralism. Another tradition of semiotics, independently founded by Charles Peirce, includes communicative action and the referential meaning of signs as well as significatory structure. Charles Morris (1946), continuing Peirce's project, distinguished three branches of semiotics: syntax (the relation of signs to other signs, semantics (the relation of signs to what they designate), and pragmatics (the relation between signs and their users). The semiotic and pragmatic branches restore to semiotics areas of study from which Saussure, for the sake of scientific rigor, would withdraw. Even a broadened semiotics, however, remains tied to the concept of the sign and, therefore, to one way of grasping language. The full spectrum of language studies includes other ways of seeing language, yielding other strategies of inquiry based on other units of analysis, and these must be included if we are to take complete stock of methodological sources. Three other ways relevant to our purpose are seeing language as speech act, as text, and as discourse. Each way can, like semiotics, be pursued through primary orientation to pragmatics, semantics, or syntax (which may also be referred to as code or grammar). The resulting array of language studies is charted in Table 1. The entries in Table 1 show locations of possible "intellectual booty." They could be filled with references in a systematic bibliographical re-

Table 1.1. Areas of Language Study

Framing Concept	Unit of Analysis	Analytic Branches of Study		
		Pragmatics	Syntax	Semantics
System of signs	Sign	Sign–sign–user connections	Structure (code) of sign relations	Signifier–signified relations
Speech acts	Utterance	Communicative performances and effects	Situated organization of speech acts and events	Contextual meaning of utterances
Text	Sentence	Reading responses, reader reception of meaning	Figurative structure, narrative structure, rhetorical structure	Authorial meaning; hermeneutic sense of texts
Discourse	Proposition	Comprehension of messages, information processing	Topic organization, propositional structure, coding of information	Referential content, cognitive meaning

view. However, I am not writing a treatise on linguistics and prefer to introduce references as and when the locations are drawn on. My concern here is only to take some analytic bearings.

Comparisons between the four units of analysis in Table 1 will bring out methodological issues and choices with respect to the framing concepts. Beginning with sign and utterance, the formal, abstractive nature of sign, especially in Saussurean semiotics, has been stressed previously. It stands in strong contrast to utterance, which restores to language contingencies of historical moment, social structure, and situated accomplishment. Bakhtin and Medvedev (1985) employ the concept of utterance to counter formalist methodology in Russian literary scholarship. The formalists, much like French structuralists, took linguistic phenomena (in their case, literary works) and broke them down into abstract elements between which rigorous, mathematical-type relations could be established. Bakhtin and Medvedev (1985) object that although such analysis is proper within its limits the limits cannot comprehend a literary work because a literary work "like every concrete utterance, is an inseparable unity of meaning and reality based on the unity of the social evaluation which totally permeates it . . . social evaluation inseparably weaves the artistic work into the general canvas of the social life of a given historical epoch and a given social group" (Bakhtin and Medvedev, 1985:125). An utterance is a communicative event within a social context expressing standpoint, preference, and identity. It is an address to someone within a social atmosphere of valuation.

The analytic force of the concept of utterance, especially in contrast with sign, is to place in sharp relief a choice between formal and concrete modes of language study, the former exclusively oriented to linguistic structure, and the latter inclusively oriented to performative context. Within the latter, however, a further choice is required between broad and limited contextual inclusion. Bakhtin and Medvedev's Marxian embrace of history, culture, and society is broadly inclusive, as indeed any form of analysis of ideology must be, but other possibilities exist. For example, their critique of Russian formalism is paralleled in Anglo-American literary scholarship by Stanley Fish's critique of stylistics (Fish, 1980:Chapters 1 and 10). In place of a stylistics concerned with formal structures of language pattern, Fish recommends an "affective stylistics" concerned with interpretive activities in engaging with language, a reconstruction of textually mediated language experiences. It is true that Fish relates such experiences to "interpretive communities" but these are construed as "interpretive strategies for writing texts" (Fish, 1980:14) closely tied to particular reading situations, not independently defined communities in the sociological sense, so his contextualism is narrowly defined.

Another example of limited contextual inclusion, belonging to a different tradition of inquiry but one also to be drawn on, is speech act theory (Austin, 1962; Searle, 1969, 1979a) where context refers directly to the illocutionary force and perlocutionary effect of an utterance in a situation.

In its close attention to local, scenic features of language performance, speech act theory is similar to the branch of ethnomethodology called conversation analysis (for example, Atkinson and Heritage, 1984). What it offers in addition, however, is an explicit concern for the locutionary content carried by language itself, a concern basic to our study of gerontology. For example, Searle (1979b:93) distinguishes between what a speaker means by uttering words ("speaker's utterance meaning") and what the words mean ("word, or sentence meaning") to explain metaphorical and other deviations from literal meaning. Without subscribing to the vexed notion of literal meaning, I think it vital to retain the point that meaning is constrained by structural regularities and combinatory possibilities operating in language, that there are Durkheimian facts of language to consider.

The analytic status of language has to be preserved against two reductionist tendencies: methodological individualism and collective determinism. The former, grounded in a cultural conviction that our acts are voluntary, reduces language to nothing but a means or tool put to use by individuals for communicative and cognitive purposes, where meaning is what we make it to be in personal and joint interpretive work. The very notion of use implies an active user and a passive used, which is misleading where language is concerned. Here it would be more accurate to speak of membership and participation than use. The concept of membership will in fact be central to our analysis of the field of gerontology.

Collective determinism is reductionist in that it tends to treat language as nothing but a medium in which higher order meanings (cultural values, forms of thought, ideological superstructures) are reflected, relayed, or imprinted. Again, language is rendered passive and plastic instead of acknowledged to be an organizing phenomenon in its own right. This was a basic consideration in my decision to be critically cautious of all forms of ideology analysis in seeking methods of inquiry.

The contrast of utterance with sign has identified two methodological choices so far: whether to adopt an inwardly linguistic approach or an inclusively contextual approach to the field of gerontology, and, if the latter, whether to take a narrow or broad contextual approach. Contrasts now of utterance with sentence, and sentence with proposition reveal two further choices: whether to stress an analytic difference between speech and writing, and, if writing is stressed, whether to concentrate on what is said in gerontology or on how it is said. At stake in both choices is whether to play up or play down the specifically literary character of the field, and whether, and if so, how, to make text a major framing concept.

Brown and Yule (1983:19), comparing utterances with sentences, associate the former with speech and the latter with writing: "we can say, in a fairly non-technical way, that utterances are spoken and sentences are written." So, when Harold Garfinkel required his sociology students to enter a verbatim record of ordinary conversations on the left side of a sheet and give a complete literal exposition of meaning on the right side (Garfinkel, 1967:25–30, 38–42), we can understand him to have asked for a translation of speech utterances into text sentences. The fact that the students found the task so difficult and, as Garfinkel demanded more complete exposition, ultimately impossible, suggests a radical division between spoken and written language in principles of construction and conditions of performance. One can find good empirical reasons for positing a distinctive logic of writing compared to speech in studies of religion, law, and bureaucracy (see, for example, Goody, 1986), and to these can be added theoretical considerations of the kind described by Ricoeur (1976).

Ricoeur critizes "Romanticist forms of hermeneutics" for interpreting texts as if they were spoken utterances, thus obliterating a crucial characteristic of writing arising precisely from its severance from the intended meaning of someone present: the characteristic of "semantic autonomy" (Ricoeur, 1976:75). The term autonomy does not mean absolute self-government; rather it indicates an unfastening of verbal meaning from the situated intentions of a present speaker and from dialogical exchange with a second person. Inscription gives an independent existence to messages and authorial meaning has to be read into a mute text:

> Authorial meaning becomes properly a dimension of the text to the extent that the author is not available for questioning. When the text no longer answers, then it has an author and no longer a speaker. The authorial meaning is the dialectical counterpart of the verbal meaning and they have to be construed in terms of each other. (Ricoeur, 1976:30)

The interpretive dynamics of reading a text are fundamentally different from those of understanding speech. Objectification of meaning in written form has the paradoxical effect of opening it to indefinite interpretation. If anyone might come to occupy the dual position of reader/author, in an interpretive space that is semantic rather than interpersonal and interactional, then fixation of meaning becomes a special problem. Not only are written words subject to polysemy but sentences and higher order textual entities are subject to what Ricoeur (p. 77) calls "textual plurivocity," opening them to multiple constructions. The specifically literary labors of commentary and exegesis display the distinctive dynamics of opening and closing the meaning of words that have been inscriptively estranged from situated occasions of spoken utterance.

As a final comment on Table 1, I would observe the evident closeness between the framing concepts of text and discourse suggested by the closeness between their respective units of analysis, sentence, and proposition (often also called a sentence statement in discourse analysis). This raises the strategic problem of how to coordinate the two framing concepts: which one to prefer and how to picture their relationship.

Our guiding formulation makes discourse a central concept, but there are difficulties in the field of discourse analysis that require critical caution in using it. Of paramount concern is the tendency of discourse analysis to methodically obliterate any strong distinction between speech and writing, thus dispersing the social, political, and analytic interest packed into the specifically literary dimension of discourse. The disappointing triviality of much discourse analysis when applied to socially significant texts attests to the problem. The problem itself lies in the analytic consequences of treating texts as continuations or extensions of speech. One consequence is that textual comprehension is made a function of individual deciphering and decoding, something going on in the mind, a matter of cognitive processes in psychological space rather than membership events in a language community. Texts are thereby reduced to materials processed by individual operations of referential identification, memory retrieval, sentence parsing, schematic organization, and the like, thus delivering textual analysis to cognitive psychology and missing the specificity of *written* discourse and its necessarily *collective* character.

By way of illustration I would point to the influential work of van Dijk and Kintsch on discourse analysis (drawn together in van Dijk and Kintsch, 1983). Their lists of materials indifferently lump together conversation samples with newspaper articles, textbook paragraphs, and other samples of writing (van Dijk and Kintsch, 1983:ix, 9). The methodical orientation to underlying propositions (discourse topics) expressed by sentences entails no special concern for textual dynamics as such. It is only the organization of cognitive content that matters. For discourse analysis, a text is the verbal record of a communicative act, of interest for what is recorded in it, for what it contains in the way of semantic information, and how that information is organized for someone processing it. Such considerations are important and we will have occasion to draw on discourse analysis in examing how gerontology represents "the" world in repeated topical structures, but we must not ignore the status of sentences as events in a reading experience over and above their discursive content. The great contribution of literary analysis to language studies, related obviously to its aesthetic interest in artefactual compositions, is to explicate the extradiscursive features of written language. The concept of text in literary theory is valuable in preserving these features, thus defending against the reduction of a field of discourse to nothing but its propositional content and structure. It is doubly valuable in specifically associating texts with writing, thus resisting tendencies to treat writing as only an adjunct or continuation of speech. To treat a passage of speech as a text or text as speech risks analytic obliteration of the phenomenon at hand. A field of discourse is a literary and textual, not an oral, phenomenon.

ANALYTIC GUIDELINES

The preceding comments on Table 1 yield a preliminary set of guidelines for our approach to the field of gerontology:

1.   To grasp the nature and significance of gerontology it is necessary to stress that it is not only a field of study (a discourse on reality) but a literary phenomenon informed by definite rules of writing that are crucial to its identity. Accordingly, the literary idea of a text will be used as a framing concept. The text–reader circuit will be emphasized to sustain the principle that writing and speech are fundamentally distinct forms of language. Not only are they governed by different conditions for achieving effects of reality, knowledge, and rationality but, as I have argued at length elsewhere (Green, 1983), the syntactic conditions of rational representation in writing are contradictory to those of normal speech and require their systematic negation. This is of the utmost importance for understanding government, bureaucracy, and the political significance of social science and other policy relevant writings.

2.   It would be as false to gerontology to treat it as nothing but a literary phenomenon as to treat it as nothing but a propositional discourse, therefore a joint text–discourse framing concept is called for. Recalling, however, Ricoeur's observations on the prospective unsettlement of meaning induced by the textual separation of words from dialogical contexts of use, we should not expect a comfortable correlation of text with discourse. Discipline discourse is oriented to cognitive integration and verbal stability but the fact of inscription means that every discursive proposition is simultaneously a textual event beset, therefore, by immanent interpretive openness. In this respect text and discourse are two poles of language between which there is a dialectical struggle of integration and dispersal, settlement and uncertainty. The operation of this struggle in gerontology will be a major theme in the analysis.

3. Language studies vary between extremely close, usually technical attention to isolated linguistic data and inclusively contextual comprehension. My guideline here is to prefer analytic inwardness, focusing on text, intratext, and intertext before—and then cautiously—introducing contextual and external factors. This is because as readers, ordinary and academic, we are so used to reading a text for something else (real world events, instruction, cultural values, ideological influences, mental states) that it takes a deliberate analytic effort to hold a text as such in focus. Application of extrinsic interpretive categories (for example, those of Marxian, psychoanalytic, or feminist theory) directs inquiry around, behind, and before a text rather than into it. I do not want to say there is nothing outside the text but the slogan is a useful heuristic device to resist our overwhelming prejudice to read a text as something else. On this point I endorse the warning and advice of Peter Goodrich:

> If the term discourse is to avoid becoming no more than a catchphrase for the textual character of ideology, it is indisputably necessary to examine how it works *as discourse*, as a *linguistic practice* or as the taking up of a position *in language*. (Goodrich, 1987:168)
>
> Rather than starting from an analysis of ideology and then reading the structural categories of legal ideology into the legal text, it is more consistent, more accessible and less arbitrary to begin with the text itself, and to analyse the specific linguistic devices whereby choices, readings and meanings are engendered. (p. 182)

Drawing together the analytic guidelines, my formulation of intent can be rephrased to state that gerontology will be approached as a field of discourse embodied in texts and realized in reading effects.

SALIENT FEATURES OF THE FIELD

To complete the introduction, I will review some surface features of gerontology appearing in a "first-time-through" reading of the literature. These are not presented as data to be explained but area markers descriptively relevant to our main question and to an interpretive grasp of the dynamics of the field:

1. *The recency and youth of gerontology*. Internal accounts of gerontology, even those of recent vintage, routinely refer to its youthfulness. Borgatta and McCluskey (1980:9) call gerontology "a very junior science," locating its birth in the late 1940s but observing a delay of academic recognition until the 1970s. The later date is confirmed by others (Marshall, 1980:9; van Tassel and Stearns, 1986:ix). Van Tassel and

Stearns add that the specialized area of geriatrics "is still in its infancy" (1986:80), even though it first appeared before gerontology. Novak (1988:15) sees a roughly 10 year lag between Canadian and American gerontology (to which the term gerontology always applies unless otherwise stated), so that it was not until 1980 that "Canadian sociology had begun to come of age." In the self-reflections of the field, recency is generally associated with immaturity, a characterization I will seek to specify later in terms of the language practices and literary composition of the field.

In summary, then, we have the intriguing spectacle of a young science dealing with the presumably recent emergence of a phenomenon, old age, which would seem to be age old.

2. *The multidisciplinary spread of the field.* Again, Borgatta and McCluskey offer a useful start. They ask if gerontology is a distinct discipline or "a hybrid creature of several parent disciplines" (Borgatta and McCluskey, 1980:9). In the same way, McKee observes:

> There is no single discipline answering to the name 'gerontology'. Old age is studied from the perspectives of many independent disciplines, which together make up the field of gerontology in their common application to old age. (McKee, 1982:299)

This picture of a decentered field held together only by an externally existent common object of study can be filled out in developmental terms:

> Gerontology was dominated in the first stage of its brief history by the doctors and the biologists. In a second stage a place was created for the psychologists and the sociologists, flanked by some economists and demographers. Now gerontology is at the threshold of a third stage, and a period of renewal, based upon the gathering of geographers, historians, linguists, exegates, hermeneuticists, and semiologists around problems of aging. (Philibert, [1974] 1982:321–322)

Along with the interdisciplinary diversity of gerontology goes a rapid, sprawling growth of publications (see, for example, the catalogues of specialist publishers such as Sage Publications and the Haworth Press). A somewhat rueful book reviewer observed recently:

> Even more rapid than the growth of the elderly population has been the professional literature about that population. Dozens of journals, monographs, handbooks, textbooks, and anthologies . . . are published every year, and at a continually escalating rate. (Schulz, 1989:139)

Interdisciplinary diversity and proliferating growth can be related to the immaturity of the field in connection with its youthfulness. It is said to lack, temporarily, the theoretical rigor and cohesion that characterize mature science. Lacking central government by theory, there is decentered diversity and unregulated proliferation.

3. *The strategic significance of demography in the existence and continuation of gerontology.* The strategic significance of demography is threefold: (a) gerontology's founding topic, the aged, was brought into measurable, empirical, potentially scientific existence by population statistics; (b) practically all attempts to introduce, overview, represent, review, or otherwise grasp the field in its entirety open with demographic observations on the size and growth of the elderly population; and (c) anything like a united discourse on aging depends on the gearing of diverse topics (the biology, psychology, sociology, and so on of aging) to the demographic framework of the field. The strategic significance of demography refers then to vital founding, opening, synthesizing, and connective functions in the literary dynamics and discursive structure of the field. It is held together by demographic observations.

Detailed demonstration of these points will be found in the main part of the study.

4. *The closeness of discipline discourse in gerontology to political action, moral debate, and ethical polemics.* Gerontology is remarkable, even within the social sciences, for its permeation by extrascientific language practices. Wershow includes "the struggle between gerontology as a field of scientific endeavour and gerontology as a cause" (1981:233) among the major issues of the area, and cites internal concerns about the diversion of gerontologists from professional investigation to "quasi-political activity" (p. 6). Academic gerontology has preserved the practical interests surrounding its institutional history:

> The impetus and foundation of social gerontology was established during the 1940's through the efforts of professional groups and other private organizations concerned about the implications of an unprecedented increase in the number of older persons in the population. (Gordon, 1981:229)

The most influential of the organizing groups came to be the Gerontological Society (founded in 1945), and the activism of the enterprise comes through strongly in the contributions and editorials of its official publication, *The Gerontologist.* Side by side with a humanitarian concern to serve the elderly one finds a political concern with advocacy and reform. The latter element has been greatly strengthened by the involvement of gerontology in government programs for the aged. A significant event (in the United States, the place where social gerontology first took root academically) was the passage in 1965 of the Older Americans Act and the ensuing growth of a massive network of agencies, programs, and care delivery systems that Estes (1979) calls the aging enterprise. Gerontology is a major player in that enterprise and this shows up in the field.

Practitioners themselves have connected the humanitarian, activist, and political commitments of gerontology to its scientific immaturity and so to the feature of the field noted previously, that its literary self-image persistently includes terms like young, junior and infant:

> Social gerontology has been criticized as being too concerned with practical issues and problems confronting the aged. Many gerontologists believe that social gerontology has grown at the expense of a more theoretical orientation. (Kart and Manard, 1981:1)

In similar vein, Johnson (1976:148) observes that "theory is a very small part of the social gerontological literature," following this shortly with an assured statement that "few people in the field will be offended if I describe social gerontology as being young and somewhat immature" (p. 149).

The question for us is the meaning of immaturity when applied to a field of discourse, assuming this to be something more than a matter of chronological recency and something only glossed by metaphors of youth. What is there in the discursive and linguistic construction of gerontology that allows it be called and recognize itself as immature?

The next chapter presents concepts for describing, analyzing, and interpreting a field of discourse, in accordance with the guidelines already given, so as to answer the question, What is gerontology? and make intelligible its evident features. Behind this, it should be added, and included in the idea of interpreting a discourse, is whether gerontology, as presently established, is good or bad social discourse. This question cannot be answered by looking at the aims and motives of gerontologists, all of which are good, but can at least be opened up by analyzing the conventions governing constructions of old age in gerontology, and the implications for people of being placed in and under those constructions.

CHAPTER

1

Text, Discourse, and Social Reality:
A Methodology of Analysis

This chapter presents a systematic exposition of the base concepts of the study, text, and discourse, within a methodological strategy I will call *constitutive realism*.

Constitutive realism supplies a rationale for making the linguistic structure of gerontology the key for understanding what it is, and for assessing its social and political significance, that is, the significance of what it does. Such assessment, the task of critical evaluation, returns social analysis to its contexts of lived experience, without which it degenerates either into irrelevance or harm. Constitutive realism locates the pragmatic relevance of textual analysis in the linguistically constructed nature of social reality, finding there also the grounds of critical appraisal. This basic continuity of analysis and appraisal along the plane of language reduces the temptation to introduce extraneously grounded, hence analytically arbitrary categories of valuation from religious, political, philosophical, and other systems of ideology.

THE DEFINITION OF CONSTITUTIVE REALISM

Sociologists have long hesitated between nominalism and realism in deciding the status of terms for collective structures. Either a term is only a nominal convenience and heuristic fiction (posing the threat of reductionism), or it names real entities (posing the threat of reification or misplaced concreteness). Given this choice, constitutive realism obviously comes down against nominalism. The choice itself, however, is misleading and false in its standard form, a predicament that can only be escaped by strongly qualifying the term realism. This can be seen by close inspection of the received alternatives. It turns out that they are two sides of a single methodological coin rather than mutually exclusive options.

The coin itself I would call substantialist realism. Reality is conceived as a substance, perhaps animate and organic, perhaps inanimate, but in any case something concrete and sensate. The only difference between standard sociological realism and nominalism is in where the substantialist accent of reality is placed. In the former, it is placed on transindividual structures existing in society, culture, and history; in the latter, it is placed on individuals and their observable actions. The position taken by constitutive realism is that where social reality is concerned any substantialist image is wrong, regardless of where it is projected. The appropriate question is not where is social reality located and in what entities but how is social reality achieved, produced, or constructed, and by what means? The reality of collective structures is that of codes, grammars, scripts, language games, and generic rules, not that of concrete entities. Social reality is linguistically constructed in and by acts of communication, especially speaking, hearing, writing, and reading. This is the basic principle of constitutive realism.

THE LINGUISTIC CONSTRUCTION OF SOCIAL REALITY

The principle does not say there is nothing outside language, which would be logically indefensible (see, Keith and Cherwitz, 1989) and experientially absurd; only that there is nothing definitely and specifically *social* outside language. (Even attributions of sociality to bees, ants, and other creatures depend on their movements having a legibly semiotic structure that is language-like: a simulacrum of society.) To claim that social reality is constructed, and can only be constructed, in language use is not to deny other reality formations around, before, and behind language. Supposed proofs of substantive reality such as Dr. Johnson kicking a stone or G. E. Moore raising his hands to audiences of philosophers (Hazelrigg, 1989, Vol. 1:457) are beside the point. Johnson did not kick a social fact, and the facticity of the supposed demonstration lies in the words representing it. Whatever realities come to us through other modes of experience they become definite social realities only in linguistic representations and semiotic adjuncts of language. Habermas, in an early, more clearly constructionist phase of his work, said that "what raises us out of nature is the only thing we can know: language" (Habermas, 1971:314). What raises us out of nature is society, and society is composed in and through language use. To language use also belong the seemingly indispensible devices whereby tracks of construction are brushed over, in passing, to leave apparently objective things externally given, for example, discourse devices that objectify aging and the aged.

It follows from the principle that social reality is made in and of language that there is no such extralinguistic thing as aging or the aged (or any other sociological category). They are *rendered realities* achieved in linguistic practices of naming, describing, classifying, referencing, and the like, both in ordinary language and specialized discourse. (The latter is our direct concern here, but its achievements of reality effects depend on continuity with ordinary language devices, a point to be explained below.) Here we need to guard against another possible misunderstanding of the principle. It does not imply a libertarian capacity to remake social reality by remaking language: idealism with a linguistic turn. Language studies reveal performative conditions of appropriateness and comprehensibility that are binding on users. For example, generative rules and deep structures underlying grammatical sentences (Chomsky, 1957, 1972), "text-grammar" rules of topical organization (van Dijk, 1972, 1977), "conventional implicatures" (Grice, 1975; Karttunen and Peters, 1979), "semantic concomitants" of words (Durgnat, 1982), semiotic structures of meaning (Greimas, [1966], 1983), generic rules of writing (Ricoeur, 1976), fields of intertextuality (Barthes, 1981; Riffaterre, 1984), and rules of local interpretation (Grice, 1975; Sacks, 1972a,b, 1984). In the present study I seek rules and necessities of gerontology binding on anyone who would enter its field, in a broad sense, the grammar of the field, where grammar means the "implicit governing practices and conventions" (Finch, 1977:158) and the constitutive necessities of a language game. (Wittgenstein's concepts of grammar and language game will be an important resource in the analytic chapters.) The principle of constitutive realism does not then say that social reality is subjectively created or intersubjectively imagined. It accepts the objective existence of social reality relative to individuals but locates that objectivity in constitutive structures of language, not in substantialist metaphors of externality. Social facts are not to be treated as things; their reality cannot be understood in that way. Neither, however, are they to be treated as mere artifacts of labeling, definitional invention, or shared imagination. Social realities are not merely constructed by language users at their pleasure, they *are* semiolinguistic structures in their own right, sui generis.

TEXT AND DISCOURSE: A DUALITY OF LANGUAGE

The peculiar elusiveness of linguistic phenomena as objects of study is evident in the protean complexity of conceptual inventions to grasp them. Charles Taylor observes an explosive growth in linguistics marked, like human sciences in general, by "mutually irreducible" approaches and theoretic warfare (Taylor, 1985:215). Yet there is in the encircling confusion one steady beacon, a repeated methodological message: concepts capable of doing justice to language must come in pairs that represent its double sidedness: the double sidedness of something whose operations simultaneously fold back on themselves *and* extend outward to things beyond—having to do one kind of operation in doing the other, or needing the absence of things to function as language, yet needing their virtual or projected presence to mean anything.

In Saussure's (1959) initiation of scientific linguistics the idea of necessary double sidedness is conveyed in the image of the front and back, recto and verso, of a sheet of paper. It follows that for every incision on the referential, propositional side of language there is a congruent one on the semiotic, textual side. The relation is not, however, quite this clear and isotopic. As Saussure explores the semiotic side of language— calling it *langue*, the code-system of language, in complementary opposition to *parole*, the individual execution of a code-system in speech or writing—it becomes obvious that its dynamics of meaning are different, even antagonistic to those of the propositional side, the execution surface, of language.

Taking the basic semiotic entity to be a sign, Saussure dissolves it into two complementary and opposite components: material signifier and signified idea. Signifiers belong more to the infolding side, the purely linguistic side, of language (just as *langue* does compared to *parole*), consequently they are for Saussure the appropriate focus of a scientific linguistics; his method moves always in the same direction. Even at this juncture there is another division and one more step toward a grasp of pure language stripped bare of discursive content. Signifiers too are doublesided. In relation to an idea they have a certain signification, something a sign stands in place of, but they also have relations of similarity and difference to each other, conferring on them a pure language value (Saussure, 1959:114–117). Thus the terms *mouton* in French and "sheep" in English have the same signification—hence their exchangeability in translation—but not the same language value because the English term belongs to an associated set (a paradigm) that includes "mutton," for which there is no equivalent in French. Hence the language values are different, making a complete, literal translation impossible. One needs to ask, therefore, of a term like "the aged" not only *what* it stands for but *where* it stands in relation to other terms in companion sets. The language values of signifiers depend on relative position in a sign system, not on necessary connection to the concepts with which they are fused, nor, of course, to real world references of the concepts.

Saussure's distinctions suggest a radical opposition between the significatory dynamics of language in itself and the requirements of discourse, especially discourse aiming deliberately for conceptual stability and referential anchorage. Paul Ricoeur nicely describes the situation:

> Language no longer appears as a mediation between minds and things. It constitutes a world of its own, within which each item only refers to other items of the same system, thanks to the interplay of oppositions and differences constitutive of the system. In a word, language is no longer treated as a 'form of life', as Wittgenstein would call it, but as a self-sufficient system of inner relationships.
>
> At this extreme point language as discourse has disappeared. (Ricoeur, 1976:6)

Ricoeur's point is reinforced in considering Charles Peirce's separate formulation of semiotics, which, even though more oriented to the pragmatics of communication, also identifies self-sufficient dynamics of meaning in language itself. I cite Peirce not only as another witness, however, but for the sake of his concept of *semiosis* to describe those dynamics, a valuable concept I want to adopt for later use. It serves beautifully to identify the dispersive strains to which a discourse is subject by its linguistic base, yet which discourse forms around and depends on to convey its propositional, referential, informational kind of meaning.

Umberto Eco makes the same point as Ricoeur, that while every act of communication "presupposes a signification system as its necessary condition," every such system "is an autonomous semiotic construct that has an abstract mode of existence independent of any actual communicative act it makes possible" (Eco, 1976:9). Autonomy is implied in Peirce's model of signification. A sign represents an object not actually present; for example, through analogical equivalence, as in maps and diagrams, or through convention, as in symbols and words. However, a sign can represent an object only for an interpretant idea (an interpretant belonging, I would say to the language competence of a speaker, hearer, reader, and writer). Peirce says that a sign brings the interpretant into the same relation to the object that it has itself, thus mediating one to the other. The crucial point is that the interpretant can enter the significatory chain only as another sign related to another object for another interpretant, and so on indefinitely. Peirce invented the term semiosis to describe this "trirelative" process of signification (Eco, 1976:15).

We can see here an inherent tension between the dynamics of signification and the requirements of empirical discourse. Peirce emphasizes that the trirelative actions of semiosis are not resolvable into actions between pairs of its elements, yet this is precisely what empirical discourse demands. It needs (and its rules of writing dictate) sign–object pairs to achieve clear referential identification, and object–interpretant pairs to secure propositional definiteness. Discursive security demands constant division and control of the trirelative process. First, to prevent a slide into unlimited semiosis where there are no ultimate interpretants to guarantee the validity of signs (in methodological terms, to dispel the spectre of relativism and cognitive anarchy), and second, to overcome the self-evident fact that signs in themselves are empty of reality, thereby threatening to rob empirical discourse of its one indispensable principle: the falsifiability of propositions. As Eco rather melodramatically observes: "semiotics is in principle the discipline studying everything which can be used in order to lie" (Eco, 1976:7).

Ricoeur (1976) articulates the problem of language and discourse in terms of a dialectical polarity between event and meaning: "all discourse is actualized as an event, all discourse is understood as meaning" (Ricoeur, 1976:12). While retaining his use of "meaning" to describe proposititional content, I will extend the concept of event to mean more than the active moment of a communication. In events of discourse there are also events of language, the self-governing operations called semiosis. There are two main events in semiosis: combination by closeness in linear chains of signs and selection from sets of equivalent signs at each link of a chain. Saussure calls them syntagmatic and associative types of sign relations: "Whereas a syntagm immediately suggests an order of succession and a fixed number of elements, terms in an associative family occur neither in fixed numbers nor in a definite order. . . . A particular word is like the center of a constellation; it is the point of convergence of an indefinite number of coordinated terms" (Saussure, 1959:126). Modern semioticians prefer to speak of associative type relations as the paradigmatic plane of language. For Jakobson (1956) this plane is governed by the principle of similarity whereas the syntagmatic plane is governed by the principle of contiguity. Jakobson (1960) took a crucial extra step in correlating these types of semiotic relations to rhetorical figures of speech (syntagmatic relations of contiguity to metonymy and paradigmatic relations of similarity to metaphor), thus building a bridge to literary theory and the analysis of written meaning. I will follow these leads in relation to the linguistic working of key words like aging and the aged in the production of gerontology discourse.

All discourse must control the dispersive pressures of language along the axes of contiguity and similarity. The demand is especially acute and performatively distinct in writing, however, due to its detachment from personal presence and immediate context. This is made clear in the problem of what linguists call indexical or deictic expressions (Levinson, 1983:45–96 offers an overview). These are terms such as "I," "you," "here," "there," "this," "now," which acquire definite meaning only in pointing to someone or something present, that is in ostensive reference to an immediate context. In situated speech virtually every utterance is a contextually determined indexical expression; in writing there is nothing for words to point to except other words and interpretive conventions of reading/writing. *The task of referential fastening passes in writing from a present context to possible worlds projected within an interpretive frame.* This point concerning the conditions of communicative sense in writing leads us back to the concept of discourse, showing in another way the dialectic of discourse and text.

Intentional pointing to possible worlds is at the heart of Frege's concept of the reference of a sentence (Frege, 1970; see, also, van Dijk and Kintsch, 1983:Ch. 4). Sentences dominated by the referential function, by that interpretive frame, are read as propositions, and propositions are the basic units of discourse. It can be argued, then, that "discourse is the equivalent for written language of ostensive reference for spoken language" (Ricoeur, 1976:88). There is, however, a decisive difference between these functional equivalents that crucially shape the dialectic of text and discourse. Ostensive reference in speech points to a present, embodied context of communication; discursive reference in writing points to possible worlds apparently transcending language yet being composed in it. In writing, language uses its own resources to achieve a self-transcendence of language. More exactly, the reality that propositions reference is linguistically emergent and immanent but in reading is effectively made external and translinguistic. Analysis of discourse must then include the literary, linguistic, and rhetorical means whereby *reality effects* of possible worlds are produced in the course of reading. Only then can it properly demonstrate how *knowledge effects* are yielded in referencing those possible worlds. The investigation of reality and knowledge effects is a basic concern of the present study.

To conclude, and accepting that "a written text is . . . discourse under the condition of inscription" (Ricoeur, 1976:23), we can say that text and discourse are two sides of a single phenomenon—written communication—operating on joint but opposing principles of meaning. Textual meaning operates on purely internal principles of sign relations (those of contiguity and similarity); discursive meaning operates on principles of external reference to translinguistic possible worlds. Internal sign relations (semiosis) composed under conditions of writing will be called *textuality.* Textuality belongs to the semiolinguistic base of discourse and must be included in a discourse analysis. As in comprehending anything linguistic, representation of the phenomenon has to be double sided.

THE CONCEPT OF A FIELD OF DISCOURSE

Gerontology is a *discipline* discourse, the foundation of a knowledge community, and as such must project a possible, investigatable world in accordance with rules, protocols, and generative formulas constituting a definite area of scholarly work. Whereas in everyday discourse the production of reality and knowledge effects is a diffuse commonplace of ordinary language, in discipline discourse it is a methodically organized expertise. I will not deny the role of ordinary language in the production of specialized knowledge [ethnomethodological studies of natural science: (Latour and Woolgar, 1979; Garfinkel et al., 1981; Gilbert and Mulkay, 1984) have demonstrated its indispensibility even there], but there is a difference and it must be marked. The concept of a field of discourse helps to do this.

French scholars have been as much at the forefront in theorizing the discursive side of language as the semiotic side. Two in particular are relevant to defining a field of discourse: Pierre Bordieu and Michel Foucault. The French term *champ* connotes a field of battle (between ideas, theories, epistemologies), a field of play (the play and interplay of signification), and a space of action and practices (practices of discourse in communicative action). Bordieu, talking more generally of the social spaces within which cultural artifacts take form, suggests that there are "fields of cultural production" providing those who work within them "a space of possibilities" (Bordieu, 1988:541). In a field of discourse there are possibilities of beginning, continuing, and concluding inquiry, of factual reference and rational demonstration, and of meaningful utterance given by shared ground rules of interpretation.

Bordieu admits similarities between a field of cultural production and Foucault's idea of knowledge formations in *The Archeology of Knowledge*, but criticizes Foucault's resistance to seeking the organizing principles of a discourse anywhere other than in its own field. Bordieu himself works with a loosely inclusive concept that relativizes discourse organization to the interests of dominant classes and their cultural hegemony in society at large, making references to their autonomy a matter of ironic disbelief (see, for example, Bordieu, 1981). On this matter our previously defended principle of analytic inwardness leads us to side with Foucault: not, it must be repeated, because of an impossible ontological claim that discourses are really autonomous but because of a strategic decision that to gain analytic purchase on a phenomenon whose linguistic nature it is to turn always into something else, it must be treated as if autonomous. Once an analytic base has been established considerations of power can be grasped as features of discourse rather than just external determinants or incidental effects. (Foucault takes this step in moving from an archeology of knowledge to a "genealogy" of power/knowledge complexes: Foucault, 1977, 1978, 1980, 1982). The remainder of this section expands concepts taken from *The Archeology of Knowledge*.

Our starting point has been the name of a field, gerontology. Presupposed in the name is the unity of an enterprise having an origin and narratable history as well as the unity of an area within a scholarly, scientific division of labour. Foucault begins studying a field of discourse by accepting such already given unities long enough to doubt them and ask "what unities they form; by what right they can claim a field that specifies them in space and individualizes them in time; according to what laws they are formed . . . and whether they are not, in their accepted and quasi-institutional individuality, ultimately the surface effect of more firmly grounded unities" (Foucault, 1972:26). For a partial answer to questions of the unity of a field, of the performative achievement of bounded organization in a system of discourse, I propose using Peirce's concept of a *legisign*. In Peirce's usage, oriented purely to semiotic meaning, a legisign is a general type that signifies by standing for replicas of itself. Proper names, common nouns, pronouns, and verbs are clear examples. All symbols are legisigns authorizing duplications of themselves either in the shape of physical, material, corporeal replicas or of other words and symbols. The term *legi*sign has, then, connotations of ruling, authorizing, governing, and ordering that I want to emphasize in transferring it from the semiotic to the discursive level of meaning. Here it can be given a narrower, more specific definition directly addressing the question of discourse unity.

I state it as a working assumption that every discipline discourse revolves around a small set of master concepts that names its subject matter. These will be called *the legisigns of a field*. In analyzing gerontology, I will treat aging and the aged as its field legisigns. They are vital in authorizing proper questions and pertinent answers, administering the orderly distribution of concepts, organizing the deployment of statements in arguments, conjectures, and refutations, and providing common points of reference and boundaries of relevance to ensure the identity of the field. Legisign replication helps explain how a discipline discourse operates as a system of bounded possibilities of meaning, such that participants can talk of utterly diverse topics yet refer to the same subject.

Field legisigns are not simply repeated, which would reduce discourse to a ritual incantation, they are articulated. I use articulation in two senses: to give utterance (as in speech) and to join (as in articulated vehicles and skeletal structures). These identify two basic movements of discourse. The first can be related to Foucault's concept of *grids of specification*.

A legisign term is never an isolated word, it belongs like every sign to a family collection of equivalent substitutes, what is called in semiotics a paradigm. Following again the principle of distinguishing conceptually between the semiotic and discursive levels of meaning, I will refer at the discursive level to a *meaning space* instead of a paradigm. The meaning space of a term includes direct verbal replicas like synonyms and (negatively) antonyms as well as instantiating replicas like representative facts and illustrative figures. A meaning space is given utterance through discursive deployment of replicas of its meaning. Foucault says that to understand the formation of an object of discourse, for example, madness in nineteenth-century psychiatry, we must include the "grids of specification . . . according to which the different 'kinds of madness' are divided, contrasted, related, regrouped, classified, derived from one another" (Foucault, 1972:42). In this example, the grids include the notion of the soul as an inner hierarchy of faculties, and that of an individual life history as a succession of phases, reactivations, and repetitions. It must be added that grids of specification need not be terminological systems or conceptual models, they can be institutional arrangements and other operational replicas of a meaning space. For example, the inmates of nineteenth-century English workhouses were specified according to sleeping arrangements and dietary lists. Architectural layouts in prisons, schools, and hospitals are other examples. They enter into discourse as operational rather than conceptual grids of specification. Both kinds are important in the emergent production and reproduction of knowledge objects in discourse.

Articulation in discourse also means to extend and link meaning spaces in a network. Base terms (field legisigns) must be turned into multiple, open-ended developments of the field. There are two major mechanisms of articulation in this sense: (1) renaming in terms of causes, effects, functions, conditions, and circumstances of occurrence, thus turning the phenomenon into contingently close aspects of itself, and (2) renaming (and revising) in terms of analogical substitutions and equivalences. Mechanism (1) corresponds to the literary figure of metonymy and, at the semiotic level, to relations of contiguity and syntagmatic connection. Mechanism (2) corresponds to metaphor at the literary surface and paradigm equivalence at the underlying semiotic level. Metonymy and metaphor are literary mediators between discursive statements of content and semiotic structures of meaning. They are, therefore, strategically crucial for analyzing the interplay of discourse and text. Metaphor is especially relevant here. Whereas standard, routinized metaphor clearly serves discursive presentation (the extreme form, "dead" metaphor, being read as literal description), "poetic" and "live" metaphor disrupts established orders of thought in writing and generates new meaning spaces open to semiotic novelty (for example, Burke, 1954; Koestler, 1964; Schön, 1979). We can see in these opposing types of metaphor a dialectic of discursive organization and semiotic dispersal. This dialectic will be examined in detail in Chapter 5.

I will take from Foucault one more observation relevant to fields of discourse and return thereby to the crucial question of their coherence, identity, and integration. He suggests that discourses exist in "systems of formation" where system means "a group of relations that function as a rule," establishing for members "what must be related, in a particular discursive practice, for such and such an enunciation to be made, for such and such a concept to be used" (Foucault, 1972:74). This idea of ruled regularity in a domain of discourse production can usefully be collated with Wittgenstein's concept of the internal grammar of language games. (Helpful commentaries drawing together Wittgenstein's scattered remarks on grammar are offered by Specht, 1969, and Finch, 1977.) In exploiting the concept, I would stress the pragmatic character of its meaning. Grammar in this sense is not a prescriptive apparatus operating over and above participants in language games (a linguistic version of normative action theory), it is more like an ethnomethodological competence to formulate and recognize meaningful utterances, an ability to continue properly in a certain way. (Coulter, 1989, offers a valuable ethnomethodological appropriation of Wittgenstein.) Pragmatic grammar consists of rules informing the moves of a language game. An observer can "read these rules off from the practice of the game" (Wittgenstein, 1958, para 54) but only because they are first built into usage. A grammatical proposition identified by an observer is a *description* of the use of signs (Wittgenstein, 1958, para 496), not a normative account of how they should be related.

Although grammar is embedded in contingent use its rules are nonetheless genuine in that they organize contingency and are not merely captured in it. Wittgenstein emphasizes the constitutive, generative, and enabling relation of grammar to practice in a way close to Foucault's notion of a system of rule in the production of discourse. For discourse in motion, grammatical regularities have the force of necessary conditions of performance. Wittgenstein says that grammar underwrites possibilities of determinate sense and "tells what kind of object anything is" (Wittgenstein, 1958, para 373). In analyzing gerontology it is important to examine the grammar of its base terms "aging" and "the aged" so as to describe the possibilities of sense they have, and what kinds of objects they are and can be in this field of discourse: "the analysis of the grammar of a word affords access to the structure of the object signified"

(Specht, 1969:184)—not, of course, the object in any absolute, meta-physical sense but a rendered object in a linguistically represented possi-ble world, which is the way all social objects exist.

I should add, to avoid misunderstanding, that no claim is being made that gerontology is a single language game ruled by one grammar. In-deed the grammaticality of joining the singular verb *is* to the convention-al name of a discourse is something that should be held in question. Wittgenstein by stressing the situated particularity of language games and Foucault by warning against the dubious unities of conventional classifications of knowledge make us wary of mistaking glosses on dis-course organization for analytic accounts of them. In this spirit I will ask only what grammatical rules or apparently necessary regularities can be seen in usages of particular concepts, not in the field as an assumed whole.

REALITY AND KNOWLEDGE IN SOCIAL SCIENCE DISCOURSE

Following one step further the chapter plan of gearing down concepts from general theories of language to engage with the particular phenom-enon at hand, I will comment on some generic requirements for doing social science discourse. It is obvious from the existence of journalistic reports, administrative documents, political manifestos, and the like that not just any organization of words referring to social life counts as social science. There is a genre-specific organization, grammar, or sys-tem of formation at work. This is no place to tackle the tremendous task of analyzing the grammar of social science, but some observations on the textual production of specifically *social* reality and knowledge effects, linking back to previous points, are in order.

Social science contains normative references to the language of its trade in research manuals, guides to theory building, and satirical po-lemics, but little in the way of actual language analysis. One of the few helpful contributions from within the field is that of Gusfield (1976). Taking his conceptual cues from rhetoric, which, with narratology, has become the major basic of linguistic self-reflection in social science (for example, Brown, 1977; Edmondson, 1984; Simons, 1989; Polkinghorne, 1988), Gusfield says that scientific persuasion rests on a "windowpane" theory and practice of language whereby it is "only a medium by which the external world is reported. That which is described and analyzed is not itself affected by the language through which it is reported" (Gusfield, 1976:16). To "do science" in writing, the literary presence of writing must be rendered invisible. Elsewhere (Green, 1983), I have reworked this idea in terms of a requirement of constitutive innocence for writing to secure effects of a reality outside itself. However, whereas Gusfield, mindful of his scientific training, is concerned with refuting the windowpane theory of language with facts of scientific practice, I treat it, via the concept of constitutive innocence, as a grammatical necessity of scientific practice: a grammatical fact about it. The language of science, at least in its authorized model, needs *not* to be seen so that it can be seen with.

Like Gusfield, I find contrast with the artful use of language in literature helpful for clarifying its literal use in representing reality. Robert Scholes (1977), pursuing the secret of "literariness" in verbal works of art such as novels and poems, finds it in an experience of duplicity in some element of the communicative act. According to Jakobson (1960) there are six base elements composing a communicative act. With writing in mind they are addresser (author, narrator, reporter), addressee (the implied reader), code (language system, genre), message (wording, verbal composition of a text), context (referents of messages, contexts of sense), and contact (semiotic channel of connection, medium of expression). Experiences of ambiguity, doubt, or uncertainty in any one element, such that simple innocence is lost, is sufficient and necessary for a sense of literariness to appear. Scientific writing, then, is governed by the regulative ideal of keeping each element basically unremarkable and free from doubt—free, for example, from suspicion of authorial duplicity, generic ambiguity, or strangeness of expression—so that reading attention is fastened to an immediately recognized referential context. An immediately recognized context is an experience of reality seen through yet outside a text, a substantive reality available for description, explanation, exploration, discovery, and other operations of science.

Immediate recognition is the key here. It is an instant fusion of reality and knowledge effects, a prereflective moment of discourse, providing a basis for secondary activities such as interpretation, revision, endorsement, and criticism. A discourse analysis must then ask how the type or genre it is dealing with—here, social science—achieves constitutive innocence in literary practice, yielding immediate recognitions of reality in being read. A full answer is beyond my scope but I will identify a major mechanism for present investigation.

The clue to identifying the mechanism lies in connections between recognition, familiarity, and membership of a methodological community. The connection between recognition and familiarity was strongly theorized in the early twentieth century by the Russian formalist Viktor Shklovsky to underpin his advocacy of defamiliarization (the deliberate disturbance of constitutive innocence) in art. He refers to people living by the sea who grow so used to the murmer of the waves that they never hear it. Comparably, "we scarcely ever hear the words which we ut-

ter. . . . Our perception of the world has withered away; what has remained is mere recognition" (in, Ehrlich, 1965:150–151). Closer to our
theme, Shklovsky talks also of reading: "reading the proofs of a book
written in a language we know well it is only with difficulty that we can
make ourselves *read* the words, and so pick out the misprints, instead of
simply taking the text for granted in an unthinking and immediate recognition of the words expected" (Heath, 1972:151).

Shklovsky's reference to "a language we know well" implies dependence of the recognition effect on membership of an interpretive community. This is brought out more clearly and narrowly in Patrick Heelan's
argument that even natural science observation is at heart a hermeneuti-
cal reading of semiotic materials: "all knowledge is *in some way* a reading
of some text or text-like material" (Heelan, 1983:184). In principle this
opens the prospect of an endless shift comparable to Peirce's sign–object–
interpretant sign formula of semiosis. If a knowledge claim (*A*) is a
reading of some text-like item (*B*), then knowledge of (*B*) would be a
reading of its "text" (*C*), and so on without logical end. Such series are
terminated in historical communities of inquirers by a conventional acceptance that there is some ultimately existant "text" simply there, a
reality given as a ground of knowledge but not in itself accessible to it, a
contextual fulness providing referential anchorage for inquiry. (Garfinkel, 1988, refers to the contextual fulness posited by any system of
inquiry, the fulness against which knowledge is inscribed, as its "plenum." In the literary practice of a discipline its plenum would be the
ultimate reference, beyond words, of what I previously called the legisigns of a field; for example, of "aging" and "the aged" in gerontology.)

Heelan takes us further with his concept of "readable technologies."
Every knowledge community has observation procedures through
which its ultimate reality is turned into conventional symbols, thus becoming *for community members* a readable text. In the sciences, instrument readings on gauges, scales, tables, meters, and the like are examples of readable technologies. For competent members, those in the
know, a readable technology communicates meaning directly, "with no
more use of deductive or inductive inferences than accompanies . . . the
understanding of a spoken phrase" (Heelan, 1983:189). Heelan continues, paralleling Gusfield, with the observation that when signs are understood in readable technologies they cease for the reader to be objects
or events in their own right and become "more like *windows into a room
that by their* (more or less) *transparent quality give direct access to the
contents of the room into which one is looking*" (Heelan:1983, original
emphasis). Through readable technologies conceptual constructions become directly recognized perceptual objects, but only for a competent
member of a methodological community.

The social sciences have readable technologies in the form of technical observation methods; this is what makes them sciences. What in addition, however, makes them specifically *social* sciences? I would say the reproduction in writing of ordinary language methods for producing accountable order and objective reality in everyday life. That is, reproductions of folk methods or ethnomethods of reality construction familiar to the reader—familiar through membership of a methodological community with pragmatic expertise in "doing society" rather than membership of one with intellectual expertise in "doing science." Textual formations that reproduce the lexicon and syntax of an ordinary language, the compositional language of a familiar society, yield an instant, prereflective, transparent recognition of a social reality there for inquiry. To help pin them down, I propose to call such textual formations *prior plausibility structures*.

There are two general kinds of prior plausibility structure, semantic and syntactic, corresponding to a distinction between meaning spaces formed by the common content of words and those formed by syntactic or grammatical structure. Of the first kind are social types, e.g., the stranger, the miser, the playboy; cognitive stereotypes (Putnam, 1975) or prototypes (Cooper and Ross, 1975) of environmental objects; plans, scripts or frames, of social situations and lines of action (Minsky, 1981; Schank and Abelson, 1977), such as visiting a doctor or retiring from work; and "genres of cultural performance" (Turner, 1980), such as ceremonies, rituals and spectacles.

The second kind of meaning space is syntactically formed, arising from grammatical rules rather than semantic content. At the level of the sentence, for example, English syntax establishes a correlation between the closeness of signs and the perceived strength or directness of connection between the ideas they convey. The sentence *Sam killed Harry* conveys a more direct causality than *Sam caused Harry to die*, which is, in turn, more direct than *Sam brought it about that Harry died*. The effect of the syntax is relayed through the degree of closeness in each sentence between the sign representing the cause (*Sam*) and that representing the effect (*Harry's death*) (Lakoff and Johnson, 1980:131). Another sentence-level example arises from experimental studies of how readers pick out the main idea of a passage of text: "The results suggest that the initial position in a passage is uniquely important, making initially mentioned information thematically important to some extent just by virtue of its position" (Kieras, 1985:100). Sentence-level syntax is also important in Wittgenstein's illustrations of how grammar misleads cognition (in our terms, how instant recognition preempts the analysis of language and knowledge effects). Coulter (1989:61, 89) usefully recalls two illustrations. We habitually misunderstand the word *understanding* because its present-continuous tense structure is the same as physical activity and process verbs such as *running* and *cooking*. A physical activity or material process must take place somewhere. Consequently the mere structure of the word lends instant credibility to statements like "understanding takes place in the mind," and to the entire mentalistic model of understanding as something going on inside individual minds. The second illustration from Wittgenstein touches on linguistic means for objectifying concepts, a procedure basic to social science. A common form of expression is the possessive locution *I have a . . . ,* where a substantive object properly completes the sentence. When, therefore, the projected meaning space is filled by terms such as *idea* or *thought*, they are readily recognized as objective entities and thereby available for discovering, measuring, and spatial-temporal location. Textual methods for objectifying the subjects of gerontology will be an important focus of our analysis.

Syntactic structures of prior plausibility are not, of course, confined to sentences; they occur in higher order levels of discourse. Harvey Sacks, tackling the question of why, when confronted with the two sentences *The baby cried. The mommy picked it up*, we instantly recognize that this is the mommy's baby even though there is no genetive "its," develops something like a grammar of social categories. Categories belong to sets, which Sacks calls membership categorization devices. The family device: mother, father . . . baby is one example; the age device: old, middle-aged, young, baby is another. Implicit rules govern the use of categorization devices. An "economy rule" allows just a single category from a device to adequately reference a person without having to state the others or name the device. A "consistency rule" says that once a person has been adequately referenced, further persons may be referred to by other categories of a relevant device. A corollary, however, says that if a first and second category can be heard as belonging to one and the same device then they must be heard that way. This rule would be contravened in Sacks's minimalist story if "the baby" in sentence one was heard to belong to a chronological age or generation device and "the mommy" in the second sentence to the family device. So we automatically join them in the stronger, more intelligible of the two possible devices at work here—the family—and read the two sentences as a narrative of two events with an instantly recognizeable, common-sensical, connection. We read typical behaviors, typical motives, and typical responses into a grammatically coherent structure of categories. Sacks adds the important consideration, and one we will have occasion to return to in discussing the aged, that in any culture there are "category-bound activities" tied to membership devices that can be invoked to praise or blame referenced persons. These belong, however, to the semantic rather than the syntactic kind of prior plausibility structure.

Stories or, more inclusively, narratives form a major prior plausibility structure in the syntax of ordinary language. Any content couched in that form will thereby receive an endownment of ordinary human intelligibility and instantly recognized credibility. Mass media analysts have become critically interested in the extent to which news reporting, especially on television, has become tied to narrative presentation. (A good, short overview is provided by Bird and Dardenne, 1988.) Part of the perceived harm to good journalism lies in the very strength of the credibility effect conferred by narrative structure and its tendency to chase out methods of reality representation directed to factual chronicling and nonnarrative (causal, functional) explanation:

> Chronicling . . . cannot fully explain and make things seem 'real' because it lacks comprehensible narrativity . . . journalists know that events seem more real to readers when they are reported in story form. (Bird and Dardenne, 1988:82)

The issue of appropriate ratios between narrative and other accounts of reality arises also in fields of social science. Here it is correlated with conflict between humanistic and scientistic ideals of discourse. The most human of the human sciences is history, and its humanistic cast is directly related to a relatively high reliance on narrative accounting. Habermas argues that historical descriptions are generically bound to the frame of narrated stories and so to the "intuitively mastered system of concepts" known through social membership rather than professional expertise, a competency shared with all other adult members of the historian's society (Habermas, 1979b:8). By the same token, however, history is the least scientific of the human sciences; the most scientific is probably economics, the one least tied to narrative explanation. In any case, there is a struggle between regulative ideals of humanistic meaning and scientific rigor played out within as well as between disciplines that, at the level of literary practice, is revealed in a competition of narrative and nonnarrative methods of representing reality. Narrative accounting is a significant feature of any field of social science, telling much of the texture of a field. As soon as a social science text seeks to show the human significance of its materials, narrative must be introduced. Connections between actants and events must take the form of ordinarily understood springs of conduct rather than causal compulsions and functional imperatives. The characteristic narratives of a field are basic textual methods of fashioning a readably human discourse on social reality. And, since narrative explanation strains against deductive, covering-law explanation, the specific literary contours of conflict between narratively and "scientificity" in a particular field are also to be included in its texture.

I have taken time to distinguish between semantic and syntactic (or grammatical) prior plausibility structures. I would like to stress again, however, their common role in yielding fused reality and knowledge effects for members of an ordinary language community. Such effects occur in the reading process each time a prior plausibility structure is textually encountered. Through them a recognition of objective social reality is conveyed. The possibility of encountering social objects is not given by our sensorimotor apparatus, which at most gives us semiotic materials to interpret, but by cultural membership and grammatical competence in language games:

> We may feel that an elephant is obviously a 'thing in the world' and that any people first coming upon elephants will give that species a distinctive name. But we will not feel the same security about stepsisters or trumps or mistakes. It is difficult to imagine human beings lacking such concepts one day happening upon a stepsister or a mistake and then giving the phenomenon a name . . . actions and relationships and feelings and practices and institutions do not walk up to us like elephants and stand there, gently flapping their ears . . . waiting to be inspected and named. (Pitkin 1972:114–15)

There is no question of denying objective social reality, only of specifying how it is objective. The answer proposed here follows the ethnomethodological track in pointing to locally organized, situationally performed language practices, but is more careful than ethnomethodology in separating written from spoken reality construction. A field of discourse such as gerontology consists of organized language practices textually performed in reading and writing.

SOCIAL SCIENCE DISCOURSE AND ORDINARY LANGUAGE

As a concluding methodological topic I will turn directly to the question of what makes a social science legibly scientific, confining attention to linguistic considerations. My major point is that although social science needs transparent continuity with ordinary language to provide intuitive contact with social realities transcending discourse, it also requires methodical discontinuity from ordinary language, rubbing against its grain.

One good linguistic reason for this is provided for us by Greimas (1987:Ch. 11). At the heart of every natural language, beyond technical and specialized vocabularies, there is a basic lexicon of around a thousand words. Its operations are characterized by protean openness to nuance, inflection, contextual variation, and the stretching processes called semiosis. All of which is contrary to the standard scientific program of cumulative knowledge through collective testing, which requires a high degree of linguistic stability, conceptual precision, and exact repetition across varied contexts. This program, worked up from a positivist metatheory of science, has, it is true, suffered prolonged assaults from several directions, but it remains the effective standard in fields of empirical social science such as gerontology. Moreover, even some of the attackers, for example, those subscribing to critical theory, share the view that nothing worthwhile can be achieved except by taking strong conceptual hold of what passes for knowledge in everyday society and its operative institutions.

This points to a second reason for discontinuity with ordinary language. If there is to be anything for social inquiry to do, faults must be supposed in prevailing beliefs: gaps, errors, contradictions, disorganized proliferation, ambiguity, and the like. If the concepts and theories embedded in social life were sufficient to understand it then inquiry would be reduced to a straight transcription of membership knowledge and social science would not be present. Research into social life, and here I am thinking particularly of sociology and anthropology, cannot proceed without taking account of knowledge structures already built into members and their ways of life. But the process of taking account cannot stop at mere collection; there must also be sorting, selecting, appraising, collating and the like. At the very least there must be an unfolding of the meanings folded into a collection of information.

Discontinuity, however minimal, with the ordinary language of everyday society implies a separation between levels of knowledge. Every social science text linguistically enacts such a separation. This is most marked in positivist sociology where the postulate of a single reality external to thoughts and words about it implies an open competition to arrive at the single true knowledge of it—that is, open to competitors meeting formal standards of logic, objectivity and testability. By definition, only knowledge statements cast in the form of what the language theorist Kenneth Pike (1954) called "etic" categories qualify; "emic"-type statements are automatically suspended. Etic statements are made from an outsider standpoint of observation and discovery, and emic statements from an insider standpoint, that of a member. The subordination of emic to etic categories is illustrated, for example, in cross-cultural studies of disturbed behavior.

Western psychiatrists have become interested in anthropological claims that there are disorder syndromes identified in folk medicines that have no counterpart in Western classifications of illness; in short culturally specific mental illnesses. The *latch* syndrome in Malaysia, the *koro* syndrome in Southeast Asia, and the *windigo* psychosis in the Northern Algonkian Indian peoples are frequently cited cases. A collection of papers edited by Simons and Hughes (1985) examines the knowledge status of such emic categories. Hughes's introduction sets a nicely etic tone in observing that the most comprehensive, authoritative classification of mental disorders in existence (DSM-III: The Diagnostic and Statistical Manual of Mental Disorders, 3rd edition) contains no entries for *latch*, *koro*, and other culture bound syndromes. Consequently, such terms belong to a scientific "twilight zone" (Hughes, 1985:3) and may distort rather than display the real pattern of the phenomena they name. To get at the substantive realities, if any, behind folk medicine terms, Hughes proposes a translatory apparatus consisting of a five-dimensional profile of symptoms and using standard description terms from DSM-III. In this way the reality and cogency of emic categories can be judged. Even contributors to the collection sympathetic to the idea of local validity for cultural members insist that "emically real" disorders must be submitted to tests of independent evidence persuasive to external scientific observers so as to decide whether they are "etically real" (Marano, 1985:429). Given the postulate of a single, substantive reality behind words and the logical inference that there is one true theory for any part of it, folk theories cannot help but be drawn into the competition for truth ceaselessly promoted by science and, since the ground-rules are drawn up by science, cannot help but be found wanting. In social science, however, where the very reality under study is made of folk theories, ethnomethods, and the like, their judgmental separation as lower, wanting, and inadequate is simultaneously a judgment of the inferiority of nonscientific to scientific forms of social life. In social science (as in bureaucratic and managerial technologies) more is at stake than the question of which theory is true. The question is, Whose rationality will prevail?

Interpretive approaches to social inquiry, tenderly respectful of the participant point of view, seek to reproduce rather than judge folk knowledge. They may even reverse epistemological authority by making members the ultimate judges of how well the observer has understood their behavior. Seemingly, even though their knowledge is separated from observational knowledge, it is not authoritatively subjugated to it as in positivist social science. The appearance is misleading, however. Authoritative subjugation is still achieved in interpretive social science but by gentler means than the discrediting, marginalizing, recycling operations of positivism. The transfer of epistemological authority to members is selectively conducted by the inquirer for research purposes, and whatever understanding appears has to be translated into terms possessed by the inquirer's lay and professional audiences. The place where understanding is effected is a text in a field of discipline discourse, conferring, whether wanted or not, a strategic power of articulation and interpretation on the author (including the author–reader as well as the author–writer). The analytically (and textually) separated knowledge of members is *made* a focus of understanding, *given* a voice it would not otherwise have, and articulated in discipline recognizeable terms they would not recognize. Even in the most sensitive interpretive social inquiry, then, there is a separation of members' knowledge from discipline knowledge and a linguistic organization of lower to higher levels of inclusion: a hierarchy of language practices.

The preceding discussion suggests there are at least three strands of language in the texture of social science discourse: an analytic vocabulary, disciplinary or interdisciplinary; ordinary language (especially the semantic and syntactic commonplaces functioning in texts as prior plausibility structures); and the interpreted rewordings and analytic remainders of ordinary language produced by disciplinary inscription on it.

An analytically defined subject matter brings into play a relevant range of theories, categories, scripts, frames, and schemata couched in ordinary language. Some of these are unremarkably relied on to secure social reality-and-knowledge effects; others are selectively marked as clichés, popular beliefs, cultural myths, ideological reflections, confusions, ambiguities, and so on. Social science shows itself to be a higher order of knowledge by conspicuously transcending the mundane level of what every member pragmatically knows. The textual performance of social science demands that this be done; it is a constitutive rule of the genre.

Inspection of social science writing reveals two further linguistic strands at work in it. First, and most variably, is the vocabularies of professional, administrative, and other operative units of a society. These also transcend ordinary language but are, in turn, incorporated into discipline discourse. This strand is especially prominent in fields of social science oriented to application and action: for example, gerontology.

Second, there is a strand consisting of elaborations of cultural values: ethical doctrines, moral philosophies, and political principles. Its generic significance for social science discourse is brought out by the argument of neo-Kantian philosophers of social science such as Rickert and Radbruch that the subject-matter of social science is value constituted, meaning that social institutions are perceptible only as embodiments of values: "Law can be understood only within the framework of the value-relating attitude. Law is a cultural phenomenon, that is, a fact related to value. The concept of law can be determined only as something given, the meaning of which is to realize the idea of law. Law may be unjust, but it is law only because its meaning is to be just" (Radbruch, 1950:52).

Anyone lacking the idea of justice could not then recognize situated actions and other particulars as being the institution of law. All social institutions and patterns are, comparably, value-given realities. It follows that if value embodiment is a necessary condition for "seeing" social institutions in experienced particulars, then it must be a necessary condition for "seeing" them in the words of a text. Implicitly or explicitly social science writing must invoke a value-relating attitude in order to make intelligible descriptions of social facts; implicitly or explicitly a social science reader must do the same. This is not simply to understand why something matters but to grasp what the subject-matter is. Because of the necessary presence of cultural values in this strand of discourse I will, with aesthetic reluctance, call it culturological language. As in its relation to ordinary language, social science discourse needs continuity with culturological language to be *social* discourse, but separation from it to be *scientific*.

SUMMARY OF METHODOLOGICAL PRINCIPLES

1.   Social reality exists externally to individual thoughts, wishes, purposes, definitions, and actions, but its mode of external existence is that of generative codes and grammatical rules not substantial things.

2.   There is nothing social—no social structure, object, or fact—outside of language structures and performances. Things belonging to corporeal and material existence enter social reality as signifiers of meaning, that is to say, as semiolinguistic materials.

3.   In the linguistic composition of social reality a fundamental distinction is to be observed between speech and writing. Not only are the structural dynamics and the conditions of performance different, but the achievement of rational order and accountable knowledge in writing (therefore in textual productions of social reality) includes negations of typical features of spoken productions of social reality in everyday life. There is an inherent contradiction between spoken and written achievements of evident sense, order, and rationality.

4.   Social science disciplines are basically literary enterprises; spoken communication is secondary, derivative, and auxilliary in them. Concepts for analyzing disciplines must be fashioned accordingly.

5.   Linguistic phenomena have to be approached through double-sided concepts, reflecting the characteristic feature of language in being both something in itself (a sign system) but in use always moving referentially outside itself (a communicative system).

6. Where fields of knowledge are concerned the most relevant duality is text and discourse. A discourse consists of propositions about possible worlds (these being, at the moment of reading, recognizeably real worlds). A text is the organization of written signs through which discourse propositions are conveyed to a reader.

7. Between text and discourse in a field of knowledge is a dialect of cooperation and conflict. Conflict arises because discipline discourse is governed by the regulative ideal of precise, stable closure of meaning whereas the textual vehicle is governed by semiotic principles of indefinite association and substitution, combination and difference (i.e., by what students of sign systems call semiosis). Discursive coherence demands limitation of textual multiplications of meaning while at the same time these are relied on as a significatory resource. Analysis of a field of knowledge should not then be confined to discursive structure and content, it needs also include the textual component.

8. Every discipline discourse has to produce, in writing, effects of reality appropriate to its field. In social science disciplines they need to be specifically *social* reality effects. Discourse analysis of any such field needs then to examine its literary means for producing joint effects of social reality and scientific knowledge of it: the literary production of reader recognizeable social science in the subject matter of a field.

9. The key to social reality effects in any kind of writing is reproduction in the reading process of semantic and syntactic structures belonging to ordinary language: the production matrix of everyday society and mundane reality. Such structures are basic to the pragmatic competence of members to make passing contingencies of act and situation into signs of an orderly, accountable, observable, and familiar reality. The structures are lodged in the reader as a member of ordinary society. When they are encountered in a text, the duplication yields instant recognition of a commonly known reality, a reality readably present in the words. Particular claims and details of propositions may be questioned or denied but only against the background sense of a social reality already known. Because of their function in social discourse I refer to such elements as prior plausibility structures. Of course, social science readers are also members of specialized knowledge communities with their own language conventions and prior plausibility structures; these are, however, more relevant to the production of higher order (including scientific) knowledge effects than the primary fusion of reality and knowledge effects belonging to membership of ordinary society.

10. The production of scientific knowledge effects in social science depends on linguistic operations as well as methodological techniques. Basic here is the subordination of ordinary and other operative language practices of society (professional, administrative, cultural) to the analytic

vocabulary of a field of discourse. Subordination may take different forms: the direct form of discrediting, correcting, and marginalizing their knowledge claims; the more subtle form of incorporating other language practices as data sources or raw materials to be worked up; or the disguised form of respectfully interpreting their meanings so as to make them clearer, where subordination is performed through understanding, translating, and giving voice to other's words. Legible social science needs discontinuity as well as continuity with the embedded language practices of social life.

CHAPTER

2

The Foundations of Gerontology

Foundations include beginnings, bases, and funding sources. I am concerned in this chapter with two foundational questions about gerontology:

1. What allowed and incited the emergence of the field? How did discipline discourse about aging and the aged become possible and compelling sometime around the 1950s and 1960s? The question refers only to conditions of discourse. I am not, therefore, dealing with organizational conditions or institutional history.

2. What discursive resources does gerontology depend on to fund its intellectual operations? What gives it food for social scientific thought and sustains the production of gerontological knowledge? I have in mind Althusser's abstract model of science as a mode of production:

> In the development of an already constituted science, the latter works on a raw material (Generality I) constituted either of still ideological concepts, or of scientific 'facts', or of already scientifically elaborated concepts which belong nevertheless to an earlier phase of the science (an ex-Generality III). So it is by transforming this Generality I into a Generality III (knowledge) that the science works and produces. (Althusser, 1969:184)

The means of production (Generality II) consist, according to Althusser, of models, typologies, operational definitions, and the like.

The economic metaphor is insightful. Also, I endorse Althusser's insistence that the "raw materials" of a science are never epistemologically or ontologically raw, never an immediately given perception of reality, but always something already worked up and meaningful. However, in view of our methodological principles, Althusser's exclusive stress on concepts and ideas must be judged unduly cerebral. It ignores the linguistic nature of the materials, means, and results of knowledge production, the operation of literary means of production (the importance of textwork in knowledge), and the discipline-specific character of knowledge production, especially in *social* science.

THE POSSIBILITY OF GERONTOLOGY

Gerontology could not simply declare itself into existence by an act of naming. The biologist Metchnikoff coined the term in 1903 but the field did not emerge for about another 50 years. For the name to become a title of possession there had to be a prepared subject matter for scientific occupancy, an accumulation of developments in social life making it possible for "aging" and "the aged" to become the foundation terms of a discipline.

According to the basic principle of constitutive realism, the guideline of this study, the social reality of events like aging, and collective subject–objects like the aged, can lie nowhere but in the linguistic processing of semiotic materials. Linguistic processing takes place in speech and writing, hearing, and reading. Semiotic materials are any sounds, marks, motions, or sensory stimuli that can be treated as signs and contain, therefore, a virtual meaning. The formation of a newly occupiable subject matter for social science must then occur through changes in semiotic materials and in the available means of processing them.

One of the few to have empirically studied the emergence of new discourses about people and society is Michel Foucault. From different parts of his work we can identify two sources of discursive novelty.

In *The Order of Things*, an historical excavation of knowledges about living beings, language, and wealth, Foucault asks us to imagine that possibilities of recording facts, posing questions, fashioning concepts, making rational demonstrations, practicing thought, and turning things into words are governed at any given time by a certain code of knowledge, something like a mode of knowledge production or a Wittgensteinian grammar of discourse pervading a period of thought, especially thought that is close to mundane reasoning, such as the human sciences. Moreover, that such codes or grammars of knowledge are subject to abrupt and total sea changes, which transform ways of seeing, and not seeing, the nature of things. For example, around the end of the eighteenth century there was a shift from seeing things in homogeneous, flat spaces structured by identity and difference, adjacency and separation, where knowledge consists of representing those relations in taxonomic grids, to seeing things in their own heterogeneous, organic spaces structured by internal rules of growth, and principles of functional connection. The advent of biology in place of natural history and philology in place of general grammar are cases in point.

A more concrete illustration, closer to the present level of analysis, is the emergence of the unemployed and unemployment as a subject–object of knowledge during the later nineteenth century. A textual comparison of the English Poor Law Reports of 1834 and 1909 (Green, 1983) argues that the unemployed was an inexpressible concept within the taxonomic knowledge code governing the 1834 report. In that code, being at work or not was significant as part of a taxonomy to classify the poor. What could be recognized as self-evidently wrong and irrational in 1834 was limited to inadequate classification and the contamination of boundaries between classes of paupers. For example, failure in legislation, public assistance and moral judgement to strictly separate the able-bodied, nonworking poor from the working poor and from the non-able-bodied, nonworking poor. In 1909, especially the minority report by Beatrice and Sidney Webb, self-evident irrationality was recognized in wastage rather than contamination, that is, the wastage of individual productive powers within the context of a national economic system. Accordingly the remedies did not lie in more rigorous methods of classification but in restoring functionality to potential workers who were outside the workforce: using test records and examination sheets to assess capacity, motivation, and potential, assigning individuals to training establishments, and improving the functional unity of the employment market through labor exchanges. Only by seeing individuals as functional entities within a higher order functional entity did discourse about the unemployed and unemployment become possible.

One source of discursive novelty consists then of epistemic breaks and transforms. These do not, of course, have to be attributed purely to knowledge codes. David Fischer, for example, describing changes in American age relations from seventeenth-century veneration of the old to phobic antagonism and the cult of youth in the twentieth century, attributes them to "a fundamental change in world culture" (Fischer, 1978:77) associated with an assortment of demographic, economic, political, aesthetic, and ethical changes. I will, however, avoid such loosely inclusive contextual accounts of epistemic change because they threaten loss of analytic coherence. Fischer himself becomes lost for analytic words. He comes to call the change in age relations "mysterious in origin," comparing it to "one of those powerful Pacific waves the Japanese call a *tsunami*" and concluding that "a great historical wave was set in motion two hundred years ago by a mysterious disturbance hidden beneath the surface of events" (Fischer, 1978:113, 114). My plan is to start at the surface of textual events and limit deeper exploration to analytically congruent features of language and discourse, including discontinuities and sea changes in them. Let us say, then, that cultural coding discontinuities are one source of new social discourses.

A second source of discursive novelty is suggested in other parts of Foucault's work, for example, in *Discipline and Punish*. Here Foucault investigates the complicity of knowledge and power, exploiting the "political" connotations of discursive terms such as grasping, holding, inspecting, viewing, aggregating, and dividing. These are more than metaphorical similarities; knowledge and power coalesce in the observational techniques of medical, military, penal, educational, and other disciplinary institutions. Speaking of institutional files in the eighteenth century, Foucault speculates:

> Is this the birth of the sciences of man? It is probably to be found in these 'ignoble' archives, where the modern play of coercion over bodies, gestures and behaviour had its beginnings. (Foucault, 1977:191)

Whereas Foucault's reference to "coercion" points analysis toward the extradiscursive underside of of the power/knowledge duality, I want to face the opposite direction—the direction faced by Foucault in *The Archeology of Knowledge*. Consequently, I would say "discipline" instead of "coercion" and stress its cognitive connotations. Moreover, I would ask *what* is playing on the embodied being and behavior of those subject to discipline. The answer, according to my methodology, must be a play of language: institutional categories, nomenclatures, descriptive protocols, case paper formats, diagnostic and prognostic schemata, etc. These methods make known individuals, populations, and behaviors contribute to the formation of human sciences not simply by providing archival data but by linguistically thickening an area of social life to a point where it can invite and support scientific colonization, that is, become a subject matter. Every science of social reality is a secondary, and higher order, reworking of a reality linguistically composed. Its possibility depends, therefore, on prior language practices grown dense, complex, and folded back on themselves.

Drawing together these Foucauldian themes, I will advance two arguments concerning the possibility of gerontology. First, that it was founded on a newly dense multiplication of meanings around "aging" and "old age," relayed through diverse, but connected, institutional language practices. (These must in modern society include mass media circulations of language as well as the kinds of practice discussed by Foucault.) A familiar phenomenon—growing old—was rendered sufficiently opaque and complex to become a subject of inquiry.

My second argument is that cultural coding problems arose in processing semiotic signs of old age (biological, behavioral, and institutional signs), making it difficult to readily read what they signified. In such conditions, deliberate parsing—the task of social science—is called for, to make a legible phenomenon of aging. Here it is worth recalling Francis Bacon's concept of science as making experience literate. Bacon, like Foucault, drew power, knowledge, and writing into a single circuit. Bacon says that experience "confounds men rather than instructs them" until she has "learned her letters," a tuition possible only in writing: "when this is brought into use, and experience has been taught to read and write, better things may be hoped" (cited in Reiss, 1982:202). Of course not just any form of writing will do. Bacon was sensitive to the fact that experience comes to us through natural language rather than direct perception, so the task of making it literate is one of correcting and replacing the vagaries of natural language with methodically regulated, orderly, cumulative discourse:

> The nature of words, being vague and ill-defined, is another source of illusion, nay, almost of violence to the human understanding. Words are a kind of currency, which reflect vulgar opinions and preferences, for they combine or distinguish things according to popular notions and acceptations, which are for the most part mistaken or confused. (cited in Reiss, 1982:208)

In today's culture we talk of educational mastery more circumspectly, and no one could unselfconsciously code the theme in terms of feminine experience being made literate by, presumably, masculine inscription. Nevertheless, if social experience is already coded in ordinary and institutional language practices, then the scientific project of making experience literate must depend on illegibilities and incoherencies seen in those practices from a more methodical standpoint, itself linguistically formed. Mastery of experience is enacted in social science through parsing language performances from social life and showing the errors, shortcomings, and infelicities found there. Cultural coding problems confer marked illegibility on particular areas of social life and so prepare sites for social science to occupy. Growing old and being old became such an area in modern societies. When aging could no longer be adequately comprehended by ordinary members' methods, and was no longer, therefore, an ordinarily legible phenomenon, it became a possible and compelling object for metamembership knowledge, that is, social science. It was not such an object for classical sociology, a fact noted by Streib (1985), who says the neglect of the topic by theorists like Marx and Weber is understandable because "during their lifetime the growing significance of aging and the age structures was recognized by very few" (Streib, 1985:342). I would add that the phenomenon was not then recognizable as a social science problem because it was still so readily recognized in mundane knowledge, still embedded in taken-for-granted familiarity.

SEMANTIC DENSITY AND THE RECENT VISIBILITY OF THE OLD

The two arguments I have sketched above are responses to the problem of recency: how it is that the old so recently became visible and how this new social category came to be formed. The recent visibility of the old is frequently noted in gerontology but not often analyzed. Typically the problem is glossed in metaphors of eyesight defects or else turned into a narrative of ideas. For example, Gerald Grob, wondering about the neglect of the lives of the elderly in social history, says: "Perhaps their relatively small numbers before the end of the nineteenth century caused them to be overlooked; perhaps the preoccupation of historians with other social groups led to the neglect of the history of the aged" (Grob, 1986:33). A typical illustration of narrative glossing is offered by Hareven: "The emergence of old age as a distinct stage of life was shaped by a larger historical process involving the segmentation of the life process into socially acknowledged stages: childhood, adolescence, youth, middle age, and old age" (Hareven, 1986:112). A different kind of explanation, the one advanced here, is that old age became a markedly visible phenomenon, hence a virtual object of study, through the growth of a dense, multistranded semantic network around the term and synonyms for it.

Identification of the strands involved is not difficult; they are evident in the textual surface of gerontology and named in its self-reflections. Two primary strands extend from census enumerations and medical science. Others are spun from the language practices of philanthropy, public care, economic management, and actuarial calculation. In all cases the strands are significantly thickened when turned into legislative, administrative, and judicial categories. I will briefly illustrate these points but not pursue the historical inquiries into the origins of gerontology that they provide for. I am asking what gerontology *is*, locating questions of possibility in the *present* organization of the field and its conditions of production and reproduction, not in past roots. I refer to these antecedents only because they are preserved in present features of the field, for example, its hybrid mixture of disciplines, applied orientation, scientific immaturity, and dependence on demography for conceptual articulation. These are matters to be explored subsequently in close readings of the field and only prepared for here.

Therapeutic treatments of the aches and pains of aging bodies, together with practical concerns to prolong or restore youthful vitality are as old as human culture. However, something new began to develop in the eighteenth century, the application of scientific observation to aging. On the one hand, the collection of statistics on age-specific death rates, life expectancy, diet, illness, etc., and on the other hand, a more systematic study of individual patients in medical practice developed. The latter development was significantly advanced in the nineteenth century when medical attention to regimens of health, anchored in the ancient metaphor of the body as a container of a certain amount of vitality that diminishes over the lifespan, was supplemented by clinical attention to organs, cells, and tissues in aging bodies. At the forefront were French clinicians of the Paris school of medicine studying age-specific pathologies among aged paupers confined to hospitals for the poor, like Bicêtre and Salpêtrière, which provided "captive subjects of long-term scientific inquiry" (Haber, 1986:71). They broke down the generalized notion of senescence as depleted vitality into particular conditions of kidneys, arteries, bones, eyes, muscles, and so on, each with a specifiable etiology and prospective treatment.

Thus the corporeal old became newly lodged in a scientific clinical vocabulary of description, diagnosis, and prognosis, and a new medical field could be imagined. Just as there was specialized treatment of the diseases of the young in pediatrics, so there could be a parallel field for the diseases of the old. Nascher (1909) formalized the possibility in his proposal for a specialty to be called geriatrics. There was, however, a basic flaw in the parallel with pediatrics that spoiled the prospects of the new field (Haber, 1986). Whereas young bodies are developing toward normal maturity so that there are clear standards of health and pathology, old bodies are changing from maturity to death, consequently the anatomical signs of diseases of old age are virtually indistinguishable from the signs of old age itself. Geriatrics became subject to a depressing tautology: "aging had become defined as a progressive disease that caused a multitude of physiological and anatomical changes. Growing old was itself the source of the inevitable organic alterations known as old age" (Haber, 1986:76). The notion of a healthy old age was erased in this mode of discourse:

> Viewing senescence from a pathological perspective, they described the entire stage of life as one long progressive disease. (Haber, 1986:67)

Small wonder, then, that geriatrics failed to take root: its idea of old age as a progressive disease runs counter to the progressive doctrine that there is a rational solution to every problem. It is culturologically unacceptable in the culture of modern societies. However, in spite of the institutional failure of geriatrics, a medical discourse of hopeless pathology was added to that of hopeful regimens of health and became part of the linguistic groundwork appropriated by gerontology as its subject matter. I would add here, further to the contravention of progressive optimism, that death is its ultimate mockery—a topic that rational discourse cannot absorb. It is one that, as will be detailed later, is important to the discursive organization of gerontology. At this time, I wish to point out only that it joins the strands of medical science and population studies in the pretext of the field.

The joint can be seen in medical statistics on populations and the conclusions drawn from them. Observers could read in the statistics the effects of nineteenth century advances in public health, hygiene, the prevention of infant mortality, the cure of diseases, and so on, such that fatal illness became more and more a phenomenon of old age: "As mortality rates dropped in childhood and the middle years of life, old age became more closely linked with death" (Fischer, 1978:108). In linguistic terms old age moved closer to death in the semantic network woven around aging. This metonymic shift gave old age a different linguistic value: "Death is one thing that has given old age a bad name. Pretty near all dying is now done by the elderly—a very recent change" (Loeb and Borgatta, 1980:197).

Population statistics connect also to the other strands of the groundwork of gerontology: economic planning, public care, fiscal management of private and state budgets, and legislative action. Foucault comments:

> One of the great innovations in the techniques of power in the eighteenth century was the emergence of 'population' as an economic and political problem: population as wealth, population as manpower or labor capacity, population balanced between its own growth and the resources it commanded. (Foucault, 1978:25)

It may be, as Foucault argues, that sexual behavior was the heart of the political problem of population husbandry, but age was the essential category for taking stock and measuring the dimensions of population. Through calculations of age-specific rates of births, deaths, marriages, illnesses, fertility, life expectancies, and so on, a population could be made known as an organic entity with its own demographic laws of growth and decline, vitality and depletion. Crucially for the foundation of gerontology, successions of census figures and running records of births, marriages, and deaths made legible a new phenomenon: the aging of whole populations. Not until population aging could be "seen" in statistics and made a visible political problem could individual aging be made a coherent object of *social* science. In analyzing the organization of the field (here and again in Chapter 5), I will argue that it is the topic, the legible phenomenon, of population aging that allows the tremendous diversity of aging—personally experienced, medically defined, institutionally defined, and culturally defined aging—to be gathered into a single, cogent object of discourse: the aged. Gerontology works between individual and population aging but is founded and depends for its coherence on the latter. It is the quantitative basis for turning references to experienced, institutional, and cultural signifiers of aging into the

standard product of gerontology: scientifically formed statements of social knowledge about aging that have public policy relevance.

An illustration of this point can be found in recent theorizing about
"the Third Age" (for example, Laslett, 1989). In individual experience,
the concept has a meaning of the kind made culturally familiar by Shake-
speare in the seven ages of man speech by the melancholy Jaques:

> First comes an era of dependence, socialization, immaturity and educa-
> tion; second an era of independence, maturity, responsibility and earning;
> third the era which is our particular topic, and fourth an era of final
> dependence, decrepitude and death. (Laslett, 1987:134–135)

However, the Third Age is not just a personal experience because it
depends on collective circumstances of work, health, wealth, and leisure. It is, therefore, "an attribute of a population, indeed of a nation, as
well as of particular men and women" (Laslett, 1987:135). At the collective level, turning personal experience and culturological knowledge
into social science, is population aging:

> A Third Age Indicator (3A1) is then suggested, expressing the probability
> of a person of 25 years attaining 70 years. The Third Age is defined demo-
> graphically in a two-fold way, as a condition of a population in which the
> general expectation of living from 25 to 70 is 0.5 or over for men, and so
> more for women, *and* of 10% or more of the whole population being over
> age 65. (Laslett, 1987:133)

The demographic condition is made policy relevant through representing the Third Age not only as a biographical stage of life and a
population characteristic, but as a new collective actant that disturbs or is
exorbitant to existing cultural codes and the institutional provisions
based upon them:

> We shall assume here that the Third Age becomes a possibility only when
> every citizen can be reasonably sure at the onset of the Second Age that
> there will be a Third Age for him or for her. By reasonably sure we mean
> two things. One is having more than a 50% chance of surviving long
> enough, the other is that there should exist a large enough community of
> those experiencing the Third Age as a phase of life, a community consist-
> ing, that is to say, for the most part of the retired, to give them collectively
> a sufficient weight in the society. (Laslett, 1987:137)

The novel actant in modern demographic times consists of active and
financially comfortable retired people. A collective form of aging that
escapes standard codes whereby retirement is placed near poverty, disability, and decrepitude (thus making the end of the Second Age coin-

cide with the onset of the Fourth), and, in escaping them, turns once valid interpretive devices into rigidly hostile stereotypes ("ageism"). By extension, institutional practices based on such codes are rendered obsolete, precipitating policy analysis and a search for institutional innovations. Medical diagnosis of aging as an illness becomes untenable; mandatory retirement at a fixed age becomes questionable; financial provision for a long, active retirement via private and/or public pension schemes becomes pragmatically significant, as do health insurance and other provisions for care and welfare. The persistance of Second Age/Fourth Age cultural codes in the context of Third Age emergence creates what Laslett (p. 156) calls "social opacity," a visual metaphor for what we are calling illegibility or lack of grammatical clarity.

From the example of Laslett, it is evident that a demographically founded narrative of population aging is capable of knitting together all the linguistic strands preforming the subject matter of gerontology. A little more needs to be said, however, about the legislative thickening of those strands prior to their being gathered into a demographically organized field: in particular, the economic and humanitarian strands of language about aging and old age.

Legislative thickening of the economic and humanitarian strands became noticeable around the beginning of the twentieth century. Speaking of the United States, which lagged behind Western Europe in this respect, Fischer says the thought of old age as a collective problem to be solved by political intervention emerged clearly in the public sphere around 1910:

> It simultaneously appeared in the appointment of the first public commission on aging (Massachusetts, 1909), and the first major survey of the economic condition of the aged (Massachusetts again, 1910); in the first federal old age pension bill (1909), and the first state old age pension system (Arizona, 1915); in the invention of a new science named geriatrics (1909), and the first published textbook in that field (1914). (Fischer, 1978:157)

Continuing with the American case, since it was here that gerontology first took definite form, it has been observed that not until the early twentieth century did the aged emerge as a separate category in welfare programs, before then being only a category of the poor and an undifferentiated recipient of aid to the needy (Quadagno, 1986:129). In terms of our analytic vocabulary, the aged became a political legisign in its own right rather than being a semantic adjunct of the poor. Along the same trajectory we can see the significance of efforts in the early 1900s to secure pensions for the needy aged: a pension being a monetary as well as linguistic signifier of old age membership. Serious political debate began with the Massachusetts Commission on Old Age Pensions, appointed in 1907, which was, Quadagno points out, "significant in identifying the aged as a special group" (Quadagno, 1986:142). The Commission could not reconcile state pensions with prevailing values of individual thrift, filial obligation, and family responsibility, but in the course of negatively marking terms like state pension, national pension, and, even more extremely, social insurance, expanded their circulation. The same could be said of early attempts to implement state pension schemes (for example, that by Arizona in 1914, later declared unconstitutional by the Supreme Court of Arizona), which "while ineffectual, were symbolically significant in legitimating the view that older people needed economic aid" (Quadagno, 1986:143).

Obviously, legislative thickening of the care and assistance strand of talk about old age was interwoven with that of the economic strand: pensions might depress wages, industry might suffer from an increased burden of taxation, and compulsory social insurance might undermine the efficiency of a free market economy. Between 1923 and 1935, 28 states passed pension laws, but they were carefully hedged with limitations on benefits, means tests, and requirements of financial assistance by relatives. The rhetoric of pension politics was fiscal and economic as well as humanitarian.

The momentum toward mandatory pension schemes under state control continued to grow in the late 1920s, helped by declining economic conditions. As the Great Depression took hold it became apparent that the existing patchwork of state, labor union, and company pension schemes could not provide sufficient economic support for older people. By the early 1930s a compulsory, national old age insurance system was an idea whose time had come, even in some business circles (those comprising "welfare capitalism," Quadagno, 1984). In 1935 the Social Security Act introduced provisions for a federal old age insurance scheme financed equally by employer and employee contributions, and federal subsidies for state pension programs. By European standards of welfare legislation the Social Security Act was a minor reform but it radically changed American politics by making the provision of subsistence to every needy person a collective obligation:

> Once that principle was established, the practice was progressively enlarged. The Congress has tended to broaden the Social Security Act biennially—mostly in election years . . . . (Fischer, 1978:184)

The Act of 1935 made it a legitimate, open-ended function of government to care for the aged, and established the principle that a citizen by virtue of reaching a certain age has a claim on national wealth just like a worker or investor. There was a resulting multiplication of administra-

tive organizations, social welfare groups, professionals, and professional associations around aid to the aged, including in the 1940s a renewed
concern to define and encourage the study of senescent care (Haber,
1986:79–80). Biologists, medical professionals, and others concerned
with senescent care founded the American Geriatrics Society in 1942 and
the Gerontological Society in 1945. Again we see a confluence of diverse
lexicons about aging and the aged, making of these terms a meeting
place of semantic pathways: nodes of a linguistic network sufficiently
complex and interconnected to be a possible field of social science.

One more strand of the linguistic foundations of gerontology must be
described. The political economy approach to aging (for example, Phillipson, 1982; Olson, 1982; Guillemard, 1983), cleaving to Marxian theory,
picks out an economic thread as crucial: wage labor. In this context,
work and its cessation is accorded a constitutive role in creating what we
know as old age. Crucial here is the labor market institution of retirement. Guillemard advances the hypothesis, based on old age policy in
France, that the coherence of old age as a thought–object arises from
retirement:

> By redefining the limits and content of this the last stage of life, the
> extension of retirement conferred a homogeneous dimension on old age—
> namely, that of being inactive and a pensioner—whereas old age had
> previously presented the extremely varied traits of individual family heri-
> tage. (Guillemard, 1983:78)

Along the same lines, Marshall observes: "'old age' in Canadian society is principally defined as a consequence of our developing (or adopting) a social institution called retirement" (Marshall, 1987:2). Using the
same formula of an institutional construction of reality, Walker says of
the United Kingdom that retirement policies created an effective equation between old age and retirement age: "in a relatively short space of
time [since the 1930s] 'old age' has come to be socially defined as beginning at retirement age" (Walker, 1983:152).

In the United States forced retirement at a fixed age did not become
widespread until the late nineteenth century (Fischer, 1978:135). Studies
of American corporations in the 1930s show that although most did not
impose a fixed retirement age on their workers, they had informal policies with the same effect (Fischer, 1978:143). The social institution was by
then firmly in place. Its effects in defining old age and the way it was a
social problem depended on lack of pensions and social insurance programs at the time. Retirement meant for most old people a punitive fall
into financial dependency rather than enjoyment of an earned reward.
Retirement defined in that context a paradoxical meaning space combining cultural approval with stigmatic economic weakness, again knitting

together economic and humanitarian strands of discourse. Retirement, however, is only one element in the linguistic foundation of gerontology and, withholding subscription to the political economy frame of analysis (see Chapter 6), it has no special claim to priority.

In sum, there existed by the 1940s a dense, infolded semantic network about aging, old age, and the aged capable of sustaining their use as the founding concepts (legisigns) of a new field of study. In Wittgensteinian terms, the semantic pieces were in place to allow for a transformation of disparate medical, demographic, legislative, and humanitarian language games into a newly organized set of games played on the field of social science. Linguistic developments inscribed in institutional practices had given rise to aging (individual and collective), old age, and the aged as self-evidently real objects in society, thus as virtual objects of social science inquiry. Gerontology works, in its language practices, to appropriate those previously formed objects and articulate the truth about them:

> The world confronts us only within language-games and is thus already articulated in detail and ordered according to the most diverse principles. In drawing up a new language-game we spontaneously make new group formations by gathering together objects with definite features or properties. At the same time we introduce a new name so that only the objects of the newly constituted group, i.e. only objects in which such and such features or properties occur bear the name. (Specht, 1969:154–55)

CULTURAL CODING PROBLEMS

The growth of semantic density around aging, old age, and the aged was a necessary but not sufficient linguistic condition for gerontology to emerge. Also necessary, and bound up with the notion of complexity, were cultural coding problems introducing illegibility or what Laslett calls social opacity into familiar phenomena. These are needed so that significant problems can be seen immediately in linguistic reproductions of social reality, in, for example, the statements of a discipline discourse. Such seeing occurs in reflexively recognized membership knowledge (and know-how), the indispensible ground of social science inquiry. It is in significant, and significatory, problems that social categories such as the old take researchable form.

Rhetoricians think of topics as places of discourse. One of their basic distinctions is between places of memory and places of discovery. The former are topic-places where known facts are stored and retrieved, providing ready access to precoded narratives and arguments. The latter are places of uncertainty, ambivalence, contradiction, and undecidability in which unknown facts can be conjectured, invented, and hypothe- sized. The emergence of cultural coding problems around a familiar membership category renders a place of memory a place of discovery, hence a double-sided category appropriate for social research. This was exactly what happened through multiplication of medical, demograph- ic, economic, humanitarian, legislative, and administrative meanings around aging and the aged. Something previously locked into ordinary language, cultural narratives, and mundane reasoning was pried loose to become an object of reappraisal and discovery. When diversified, the linguistic course of social life gives rise spontaneously to breaching expe- riences, disruption of taken-for-granted reality, and, therefore, to possi- bilities of inquiry.

Circumstantial evidence of cultural coding problems is plentiful in the extreme mixture of positive and negative images of aging to be found in mass media, artistic and other cultural enlargements of ordinary lan- guage ways of construing old age. Fischer (1978), reviewing American cultural documents, discerns gerontocratic reverence for old age in the eighteenth century, then a transition to gerontophobic repulsion in the later nineteenth and early twentieth centuries. Such contrary images are culturally widespread and remain, in various expressive guises, in cur- rent circulation. Michel Philibert (1982), for example, arguing that geron- tology cannot escape choice between imagining old age either as a calamity everyone must suffer, a period of physical decline, mental dete- rioration, and social disgrace, or an opportunity for inner exploration and spiritual growth, draws on the most diverse sources to illustrate the two kinds of image: Confucius, the films of Ingmar Bergman, Bau- delaire, and novels by Benoite Groult, Paul Guimard, and Dan Green- berg. The list could, of course, be hugely expanded.

Closer to our interest in language analysis, cultural Manicheism about old age has been color-coded in gray and gold. Eighteenth-century New Englanders believed in a Gray Champion who appeared in moments of adversity: "But should domestic tyranny oppress us, or the invader's step pollute our soil, still may the Gray Champion come" (Hawthorne, 1987:132). In our own day, the Gray Panthers, a multiage activist group, has come to symbolize political potency in older people, as has the "gray lobby" in Washington (Pratt, 1976). Gray power also refers to the eco- nomic strength of senior consumers: "It's called the invisible market. The grey group. The new Old. In this world still awe-struck by youth, the fastest growing, richest group of people has gone unnoticed. They're over 50 Untargetted by marketers. An untapped resource" (Nesdoly, 1988). In Canada, a marketing company designed to unlock the buying power of the new old calls itself Grey Canada.

Gold is a positive symbol both of economic and spiritual prosperity in older people. An English newspaper article headed "Why Old Means Gold to the Marketing Men," describes how "grey is beautiful" and "old is gold" (*The Sunday Telegraph*, March 18, 1989:11). In the same newspaper (July 30, 1989, Appointments section:1) an article on the "industrial renaissance for the much-maligned over 50s" due to a shortage of young workers is headed "Golden Oldies poised to make comeback." On the personal growth theme, a recent look on creative retirement for older people, here called "maturians," is titled *The Golden Revolution* (Drabek, 1989). Retirement is often euphemized as the dawn of an individual golden age: a popular television series about older women is called *The Golden Girls*, and voluntary associations of older people are commonly called Golden Age clubs.

On the negative side, gray also encodes individual and collective enfeeblement. A report in the American Psychological Association *Monitor*, July 1985, on a meeting of experts on aging, says: "one speaker after another echoed his view that we need no longer fear hurtling through the years toward an inevitable, feeble grayness." The fear, nonetheless, is there as can be seen in the fact that gray hair is for so many a dyeing matter. At the collective level, phrases such as the graying of America (or any other society) signal concerns about vitality, strength, and potency, as well as about the burden of the frail, needy, dependent, unproductive aged on the working population. Demographic graying betokens crises (medical, financial, and moral) in carrying an increasing burden of old people.

Chronic ambivalence in images of aging offers circumstantial evidence of coding problems. More direct symptoms can be read in gerontology itself. Not only does it repeat the ambivalent formulations of everyday society in its depictions of aging, and rework them in its explanations (in, for example, activist versus disengagement theories—and normalizations—of aging), but its attempts to grasp the aged in methodically exact categories frequently lapse into oxymoronic conjunctions of opposites, such as the "new–old" and "young–old." Bernice Neugarten introduced the latter term in 1974 as part of a systematic classification (Neugarten, 1974). Then it meant persons who are 65 to 74 years old. Subsequently it has been stretched downward to include those aged 55 to 74. Especially it refers to the active, healthy, well-off old who defy the conventional marks and signs of elderliness: the nonelderly elderly who are relatively old in years but not culturally decipherable as old: "The champions of the new old seek to liberate older people from popular myths of weakness, disease, passivity, decline, uselessness, and other images of loss commonly associated with aging" (Cole, 1986:49). Gerontological gray champions seek then to study and help a social category from which recognitional signs (the signs of membership knowledge) are to be removed, making of it a self-cancelling category.

FORMS OF CODING PROBLEMS

Ambivalence and ambiguity have become deeply engrained in our ever-expanding ways of speaking about old age. I wish now to trace this fact to particular cultural coding problems. The discussion is guided by the assumption that cultural organizations of meaning contain general, structurally based possibilities of coding difficulties, identifying universal kinds of problems. Three kinds will be considered here in relation to aging and the aged in our society: (1) problems arising from the organization of meaning spaces around core values, (2) problems arising from the organization of meaning spaces between polar opposite values, and (3) problems arising from the latent, semiological organization of meaning spaces into quadrangular sets. This is the deepest kind in that coding problems are compounded by the fact that seemingly single core values and simple binary pairs belong, of semiological necessity, to complex semiotic squares. (The theory and concept of the semiotic square belong to Greimas; a helpful summary is in Schleifer, 1987:25–36.) Negotiation of a square is, of course, all the more difficult if one imagines it to be another shape.

1. Core Values and Marginal Identity.   A core value defines self-evident desirability in self and society. It provides obvious criteria for positive and negative evaluations, projecting a semantic network of positive and negative meaning spaces, including normal and marginal identities, together with rules for assigning individual and collective actants to them. Such rules of assignment operate almost automatically in the sense of yielding instant, prereflective judgments of worth. Coding problems arise from the persistence of moral sensitivities and ethical intuitions rooted in past core values. For example, continuations of aristocratic, rural, and Christian values in egalitarian, urban, secular society. Through such value remnants, the present casting of particular actants, say the elderly, into negative meaning spaces can feel wrong or distasteful even for those subscribing to the current core value composing those spaces and supplying the rules of assignment. Stigmatization of the old might feel wrong yet be in perfect accord with the judgmental logic of an accepted core value.

The most obvious values predefining the worth of the old in our society are youth, independence, and economic productiveness. Gerontologists describe and in various tones deplore their marginalizing effects without, however, being able to reject the values concerned. Gerontology thus explicates and exemplifies a coding dilemma built into membership knowledge.

Exaltation of youth and correlative repugnance for old age is a commonplace topic:

> We are still glamorizing youth and may still be at the point mentioned by Margaret Mead: In our society the old are strangers in the land of the young. (Monk, 1980:46)

One of the strongest statements of the point is in Fischer's history of American attitudes to aging (Fischer, 1978:113–156), which chronicles the development of a "cult of youth" from 1770 to 1970 that made "victims of the aged" (p. 198). Fischer is distressed by the results of making the old marginal and stigmatic but cannot see it as any more than an attitude problem soluble by fairer treatment, finding a pragmatic balance between extreme positions, exercizing tolerance, and seeking a liberal consensus:

> If we wish to work toward a new model of age relationships, then surely it should be a world without *gerontocracy* on the one hand or *gerontophobia* on the other. It might be built upon an ideal of *gerontophratria* instead—a fraternity of age and youth . . . a world in which the deep eternal differences between age and youth are recognized and respected without being organized into a system of social inequality . . . a system of age relations in which youth is not oppressed by age, as often it was in early America; and age is not oppressed by youth, as sometimes it is in the modern world. (Fischer, 1978:199)

Fischer's prescription resonates with culturally authenticated beliefs. He views the problem within the confines of membership knowledge and cannot, therefore, see it as a problem *of* membership knowledge. To do that requires reflexive analysis: grasping the problem of the old as one generated in certain practices of reality and knowledge production, not one given in objective reality; seeing it as a problem built into membership knowledge and its rules of production, including the limits it must place on reflexion. I have indicated previously and will argue throughout that the coherence and integrity of gerontology depend on its adherence to the basic game rules of mundane knowledge production, however much it might contest particular contents of mundane knowledge in the name of science. Fischer's text is then representative of the field in this respect.

There are two other points worth making about youth as a core value
(i.e., a primary means of knowledge production). First, it provides for
stigmatization of the active, powerful old as well as the passive and
weak. Hostile resentment rather than pitying contempt is the key tone
here. For example, a recent newspaper article polemicizes gerontocracy,
"the commonest form of government in history," warning that old
minds, due to neural deterioration, become inefficient and unstable,
threatening societies governed by them with the fate of ancient Sparta
"destroyed by the senile petulance of the Gerousia" (a governing body
excluding anyone younger than 60), or that of contemporary Commu-
nist regimes (Berry, 1990). Fischer (1978) offers comparable examples of
youth-biased resentment of control by the old.

A second point is that youth provides for a dimension of judgment,
the aesthetic dimension, not found in the other core values. The negative meaning space projected here is that of repellant ugliness. It is
present not only in advertising and the arts but in areas of interaction
such as medical care. Eisdorfer and Cohen, commenting on the disproportionate enthusiasm for child care relative to care for the aged, and the
well-known difficulty of getting doctors to specialize in geriatric care,
observe: "Older persons are often seen as generally undesirable patients
and unappealing persons" (Eisdorfer and Cohen, 1980:55). The aesthetic
dimension is also important in social work and in domestic and institutional ill treatment of elderly people.

There are two other core values making old age a marginal, deviant
social location: independence and economic productiveness. Of primary
importance in both cases is a significatory connection between want of
the value, lack of clear social identity, and loss of individual personality
(i.e., the rights and privileges of a full person).

Starting with a standard gloss: "the ethos of independence and self-
sufficiency still permeates our culture and is still a standard against
which individuals and groups often measure their own and each other's
worth" (Cantor, 1980:131). Stated more positively: "Only by being independent can an American be truly a person, self-respecting and worthy
of concern and the esteem of others" (Clark, 1972:263). Lack of independence, then, makes one less than a full person—a child, for example:
"The notion exists that every person should be in charge of him-
self/herself and economically self-supporting. Dependency in the economic sense, or even in the physical sense, is seen to render a person
childlike" (McDaniel, 1986:58).

The negative meaning spaces cast by lack of independence contain
other occupants than the childlike person, yielding further semantic
associates of old age troublesome to ordinary sensibility. These include

blameworthy failures, impotent victims of circumstance, victims of discrimination, and problem populations. I will briefly illustrate these points, leaving deeper examination for the next chapter.

Thomas Cole (1986) analyzes cultural links between signs of old age and nineteenth-century American Protestant theology, which interpreted them as reminders of Adam's transgression, Edenic eviction, and divine punishment for human sin. These connotations were carried over in the new middle-class morality of ascetic self-control: "The primary virtues of civilized morality—independence, health, success—required constant control over one's body and physical energies. The decaying body in old age, a constant reminder of the limits of physical self-control, came to signify dependence, disease, failure, and sin" (Cole, 1986:50). Jules Henry (1966) includes body control (e.g., sphincter control) among the "personalizing factors" allowing us to achieve individual identity within collective life: having to be moved, cleaned, fed, and so on is, therefore, to lose basic means of individuation and to risk losing "the right to personality" (Henry, 1966:291). In this context it is culturally logical that old people should be associated with disabled people: "After all, the blind, the lame, and the intellectually retarded are—like the elderly—victims of conditions over which they have no control, and because of which they may suffer deprivation and even stigmatization" (Eglit, 1985:538). The deprivation, however, is not just of capacities and resources but of the symbolic means for showing oneself to be a regular member of society and an individual personality.

It is also culturally logical that the old should come to play the ancient role of the goat on which iniquities are heaped. To the theological, existential, and psychological iniquities discussed by Cole, Binstock (1983) adds economic and political frustrations. Here, however, an odd dialectic develops between the old as victims of society and society as a victim of the old. Whereas the deficiencies of the old, by marginalizing the group, prepare it for the scapegoat role, the actual script includes the group's strength and activity. It is numerically strong and growing, and it is placing great and growing demands on government budgets enforced as much by its own political muscle as by the conscience of the nonold. It has become an economic problem population threatening to the social whole and liable to accusations of selfish greed or shameless exploitation.

Attributing a threatening strength to people marginalized by their deficits is, of course, a familiar feature of minority group discrimination, so it is not surprising that serious consideration has been given to the question of whether the old is a minority group in the technical sociological sense:

> In the literature on dependency it is easy to recognize that dependency is a
> specially used concept in gerontological studies. If it is not used in connec-
> tion with old age it mostly involves psychiatric patients and deviants and
> sometimes ethnic minority groups. (Van den Heuvel, 1976:162)

We see once more what estranged, marginal semantic company the
old must keep. As to whether the old is in its own right a discriminated
minority group, the consensus seems to be that the category has some
but not all of the defining criteria (Harris, 1988:117). The important
point, however, is the cultural plausibility of making the equation at all,
and the equal difficulty of being able to recognize personally known old
age in it.

Economic productiveness is closely linked in our culture to independence, and removal from it is comparably related to marginalization,
social opacity, and uncertain personal identity. People who are permanently not in work (not even prospectively as in the case of children and
the unemployed, or tangentially as in the case of full-time housewives)
are not fully in society. The economically marginal are construed as
something *on* rather than *in* society. A standard gerontological observation is that age structure—for example, top heavy bulging in the population age pyramid—has implications for "the economic burden that a
society must bear in supporting its dependent members" (Marshall,
1987:18). Retirees and old age pensioners are thus brought within linguistic range of single mothers, unemployable drop-outs, homeless people, and other financial crosses to be borne by the productive members
of society. Compensatory rhetorics of inclusion such as welfare state
rights of citizenship, or continuity with work through an active retirement, do not change the logic of marginalization dictated by loss of
economic productiveness. They may indeed deepen its effects. Morgan
(1979) argues that just as parental words of love uttered in an unloving
tone or a doctor's words of hope spoken hopelessly place a child or a
patient in an emotional double-bind, so exaltations of retirement in a
society oriented to the value of work place the retired elderly in a cultural double-bind: "Under this pervasive value structure, it is somewhat senseless to argue that older persons should find other outlets in
retirement to compensate for loss of the vocational role . . . this culture ascribes worth to a person's job role, and retirement does not
bear a positive connotation" (Morgan, 1979:38). The concept of a cultural double-bind is, then, another way of talking about cultural coding
problems.

In being economically marginal and permanently outside of work, the
aged become socially opaque:

> Work is not only the means to one's own resources, it is also the vehicle through which one contributes to the community. Leisure is somehow thought of as non-productive. (Tropman, 1987:47).ep

In other words, work (activity certified to be productive through financial payment) is indispensible for making one's membership status evident and visible; leisure activity does not produce such evidence. Membership visibility is not, of course, the same as conspicuousness. Mizruchi (1983) calls the elderly "the most conspicuous of the surplus populations of contemporary America" but alludes to social opacity in comparing the elderly, "found wandering aimlessly through the downtown areas of America's cities," with "unattached youth roaming the streets in London during the early part of the nineteenth century," on the grounds that the aimlessly wandering elderly are also "without work and without school" (1983:49).

In being socially opaque and placed in the shadowy penumbra of cultural meaning spaces, people also tend to lose individual identity, to become depersonalized:

> Since old people in our culture who have withdrawn or have been displaced from the occupational system can no longer succeed or fail, they are scarcely people at all—unless, of course, they can still symbolize their past success by continued consumption capability. (Henry, 1966:284)

Even continued consumption of status symbols is not good enough to secure full membership status, however, since it is active participation in "the war of success and failure" (Henry, 1966:285) that makes one fully visible and endows one with moral presence in our collective life. Political activity is thus the main feasible alternative to productive activity in giving signs of full social membership and making oneself count as a person.

To collect these observations on core values it is helpful to note that youth, independence, and economic productiveness all come under the general formula of American culture (which is by no means confined to the United States) that Parsons calls "worldly instrumental activism" (Parsons, 1989:595).

Parsons has good claims to be called the premier exponent of core value analysis; moreover, his formulations of a genetic relation between culture and social structure are appealingly close to our methodological position. He distinguishes delicately between individual value relations (components of personality), institutional value relations (components of roles, organizations and the operative units of social systems), and higher order value-orientations belonging to culture itself. Values are imagined cybernetically to "govern action in society" (Parsons, 1989: 583), but also genetically to constitute society. They are normative patterns existing above and prior to any particular occasions or concrete exigencies of action, being in this respect like grammatical rules in relation to language-games and possibilities of performative coherence. They involve "only the exigencies which are *generic* to the category of social system in question" which, in the case of a society, "include the fact that it is a social system at all" (Parsons, 1989:579. Original emphasis).

The defining formula of American society—worldly instrumental activism—is a grammatical definition, hence a performative predefinition, of what is worthwhile and estimable in individuals, actions, organizations, institutions, and the society as a whole. Parson's observations on the meaning of the formula can be applied directly to the marginalization of the old. First, extending the line taken by Weber in connecting ascetic Protestantism to the work ethic, he observes that a value-orientation to worldly instrumental activism dictates in practice a high moral evaluation of economic activity: "operatively the general adaptive emphasis throws particularly strong stress on the function of economics production, particularly the increase in the level of productivity of the economy" (Parsons, 1989:608). As we have seen, not only are the retired elderly individually non-productive but the combined weight of the old on collective resources is threatening to the productivity of the national economy. There are, however, less obvious implications. It follows from the instrumental emphasis that individual and collective actants will be judged by what they do rather than what they are; moreover, the judgment will depend on universal criteria of performance applied "'impartially' and 'objectively' to all units competing in the evaluative field" (Parsons, 1989:596). The old are typically on the sidelines of the central evaluative field, economic production, and even success as a consumer is only a secondary achievement. Parsons emphasizes that in an instrumental value context, economic evaluation is not primarily consummatory or a matter of hedonistic enjoyment.

We can say, then, that a chronic problem for the old is curtailment of criterial performance activities. This is not only a matter of competitive failure, as in everyday physical tasks and sexual activity, but withdrawal of competitor status and systemically enforced deviation from instrumental activism. This aspect of aging has been conceptualized in gerontology as "disengagement theory." First presented by Cumming et al. (1960) and Cumming and Henry (1961), the theory proposes a normal and healthy decrease in social interaction, and withdrawal from social roles as individuals grow old. Parsons allows the theory to be seen as a euphemistic gloss on a culturally compelled process of stigmatic marginalization. Without access to criterial activities in which to show identity and worth individuals are rendered socially opaque and morally nebulous, epistemologically blurred, and normatively dubious. Parsons reinforces the point in observing that access to fields of performance is provided by institutionalized roles in the operative units of society. It follows that role disengagement in general and economic role disengagement in particular must pose an irresolvable problem of identity and worth within the cultural logic of instrumental activism. The problem of identity is intimated in Keith's application of the idea of liminality, derived from the Latin for threshold, to aging (Keith, 1985). Liminality is a state of suspension between social positions, as in honeymooners, military recruits entering training camp, and "initiates suspended between non-membership and belonging" (Keith, 1985:254). Retirement is another case of the same state. Liminality can, as Keith stresses, be an occasion for creativity, recreation of the self, and spontaneous solidarity, but growing old in modern societies is more likely to leave individuals in a state of limbo: "The exit signs are numerous, but the individuals moving out of social participation as mature adults are stranded without a pathway to reincorporation" (Keith, 1985:253).

The dark side of liminality is brought out in the distinctions between "institutional roles," "tenuous roles," and "amorphous positions" made by Rosow (1985). An institutional role has clear status definitions of rights and obligations plus definite, substantial role contents; a tenuous role has a clearly labeled status but vague, insubstantial role contents; an amorphous position is poorly defined with indeterminate and insubstantial content. The "genuinely amorphous . . . include many who are devalued, both deviants and others who exemplify social loss, failure, stigma, or marginality" (Rosow, 1985:69). Among them are young divorced mothers, the chronically unemployed, long-term inmates of mental hospitals, and the elderly. The same kinds of life change in old age construed by Cumming and Henry as normal disengagement are seen by Rosow as role shrinkage and role emptying, leaving the elderly in a marginal and precarious position: "they are judged invidiously, as if they have little of value to contribute . . . the aged are arbitrarily stigmatized as having little marginal utility of any kind, either economic or social" (Rosow, 1985:71).

Parson's specification of core value analysis enables us to understand why as a matter of cultural logic the old are devalued, stigmatized, and conceptually associated with such strange and disturbing company. With the formula of worldly instrumental activism in mind we can understand how it is reasonable for Eisdorfer and Cohen (1980) to contrast our lack of clear roles for the elderly with the clear role assigned to elderly macaque monkeys who, being readily expendable, are posted on the dangerous boundaries of the group (a grim kind of marginal utility) and we can grasp the cultural logic they try to deny in quickly adding a disclaimer to what they might be heard to mean: "It is clearly inappropriate to amputate the aged from our society" (Eisdorfer and Cohen, 1980:66). Amputate may be the wrong word but some such term is surely appropriate for what must be done to worldly instruments that have lost all use. Through Parson's formula we can also understand why the contest posited by Philibert (1982) between aging as an ineluctable calamity and aging as spiritual growth is, in fact, no contest. As Parsons says, an orientation to worldly activism precludes "primary concern with internal value-realization" (Parsons, 1989:607), that is, with spiritual growth, and renders anything like philosophical resignation to mortality, which might otherwise be part of the wisdom of old age, a moral delinquency: "'Fatalism' both at the societal and at the individual level is totally unacceptable" (Parsons, 1989:594). Ceaseless worldly activity is demanded as much of the old as the young to be social members in good standing.

2. *Value Dualities and Aporias of the Aged.* According to standard conventions of rational thought a term such as "the aged" or "the old," a noun plus the definite article, designates a singular object: the actual aged, the real aged, and the true old. There is assumed to be a homologous correspondence between the sign and that which it represents. Postmodernism challenges this assumption (for example, Benhabib, 1984) by making inventive paralogy, against legislative homology, a principle of knowledge production (Lyotard, 1984). Paralogy includes singular terms that refer to opposite properties so that the one true nature of the object referred to is undecideable. While aporia is a virtue for postmodernism, however, it is only an illogical paradox within the still dominant homological regime of modernist, "analytico-referential" discourse (Reiss, 1982). By an aporia of the aged I mean a chronic and unsettling doubt regarding the location of the named object between two opposite value terms.

Tropman (1987:27) argues that cultural values tend to form paired sets, each set a "dualistic paradigm" involving systematic contradiction and "sociological ambivalence." He follows Erikson (1976) in taking issue with core value analysis. According to Erikson, culture includes the organization of divergency as well as consensus: "the identifying motifs of a culture are not just the *core values* to which people pay homage but also the *lines of point and counterpoint* along which they diverge" (cited in Tropman, 1987:27, original emphasis).

Applying the idea to policy analysis, Tropman emphasizes the cognitive dimension of value sets. Dualistic pairs generate opposing interpretive categories that define opposite sides on any given policy issue. The crucial point, however, is that each side relies on the negative presence of the other for its own definition. The dualities underlying policy conflicts are thus cognitively complementary as well as evaluatively opposed:

> To think about things public requires one to think also about things private; to think about family requires thinking about the individual; to think about self-reliance requires thinking about dependency. In every instance the values are locked together. (Tropman, 1987:31)

This is an advance on core value analysis in that coding problems are attributed to the very structure of a cultural code—its organization into opposite yet complementary pairs of values—not just to the content of a code, as in the evaluatively unacceptable implications of an accepted value. The next section, on semiotic squares, will carry the structural explanation of coding problems one step further. Before that, however, I will provide some illustrative comments on value dualities that confer cognitive ambivalence on the old within our members' ways of thinking.

Tropman (1987:30) lists several dualities significant for policy debate on the elderly: private vs. public, person vs. family, competitive struggle vs. membership entitlement, work vs. leisure, and independence vs. interdependence. The last pair is so basic to the field of gerontology that I have made it the subject of a separate chapter and will not deal with it further at this point. Commentary here will be confined to the first three pairs on the list.

To illustrate the ambivalent position of the elderly between private and public value locations, I will return to the argument of Fischer (1978) that around 1910, in the United States, old age began to be thought in a new way, namely as a public problem to be solved by government intervention rather than a set of contingent private problems to be solved by individual provision and family care. The coding problems thus created in thinking about the problems and solutions of old age are evident in the case of proposals for compulsory old age pensions in the early 1900s.

Advocates appealed to European examples but in the American context, dominated by values of private enterprise and individual resourcefulness, compulsory public pensions were not recognizeably rational solutions to problems of poverty in old age. They were denounced as "a corrupt form of socialism . . . dangerous to American liberty and . . . hostile to the morals of the Republic" (Fischer, 1978:168).

The issue was not, however, so easily settled. Denunciations from the standpoint of private individualism included positive thought of public collectivism under another name: the Republic. Military veterans already received state pensions, a fact exploited by William Wilson, Secretary of Labor, when introducing the first national pension plan in 1909. The proposal was to enlist all Americans aged 65 or over, if below a certain income level, as "privates" in an "Old-Age Home Guard of the United States Army," their pensions being a pay for patriotic duty in reporting to the War Department once a year. The ploy failed but the cognitive interlocking of private and public, individual and collective, rendering impossible a pure normative distinction between them, remained to be exploited again. In the early 1930s a national crusade developed around the Townsend Plan. Once more pensions were legitimated as private payments for a public service. Now, however, the service was to be economic rather than military. The elderly, called in the Plan "civil veterans of the Republic," were to be given a monthly pension on condition that they spent it as quickly as possible. Their public service was to be "circulators of money" and "distributor custodians of the nation's wealth" (Fischer, 1978:181). The Townsend Plan came to nothing but, like the 1909 proposal, its semantic contortions are symptomatic of an underlying cultural coding problem. Continuing and unresolved arguments about the proper role of the state in supplying individual wants (for example, Olson, 1982:11–21) indicate that the old remain ambivalently caught between two value complexes that are themselves ambivalently interlocked.

Estes (1979) uses dual value analysis to identify problems in the 1965 Older Americans Act and its implementation. She traces many of them to an ambiguity underlying the Act. It is informed, she argues, by two "myths" or cognitive paradigms of old age. One makes us see the needy aged as individuals responsible for their own plight because they did not work hard enough or save enough; they deserve only minimal assistance to be carefully targeted by fiscally responsible agencies under government control. The other "myth" represents the needy aged as a no-fault victim category suffering from defects built into the political economy; they deserve maximal assistance and appropriate services through generous large-scale programs. The stated objectives and public rationale of the Older Americans Act reflect the no-fault, maximal assistance myth but its implementation is structured by the own-fault, minimal assistance myth, even though it is nowhere stated in so many words, either in the legislation or its administrative documents. Estes, who has practical as well as scholarly knowledge of this policy, asserts that the legislation "actually contains a pair of opposing myths and definitions about the elderly . . . the intentionally ambiguous language of the Older Americans Act prevents both a clear understanding of the problem and the testing of alternatives . . . a contradiction of policy choice results" (Estes, 1979:30). Regardless of whether intentionality can be proved, the radical ambiguities undermining the program represent an aporia in the cultural matrix of American society, consequently the program could be called democratic in the sense that it represents popular opinion. The own-fault, individual responsibility paradigm as at least as valid, culturally, as its opposite and will, therefore, if representative democracy works, find its way into public policy.

Estes also reveals another duality, the final one for present discussion, in American and, more broadly, liberal democratic public policy on the old. Now, however, the duality is a difficulty as well as a topic of her presentation. It can be called a paradox of liberal humanism. The paradox is that liberal humanism is oriented to the unique value of each individual and has, therefore, a principled objection to placing individuals in judgmental categories, something it registers as prejudice (for example, racism and ageism); yet public implementation of the value entails action on behalf of such categories, thereby giving positive value to categorial identity, the antithesis of unique individual identity. Individuals are, in liberal humanist public practice, absorbed into protection groups, client groups, legislative classes, and administrative categories. Collective action on behalf of individual identity positively promotes its interlocked opposite, hence the poignancy of the liberal welfare state and the dilemmas of social work.

Estes touches on the problem of having to talk categorially about the old in criticizing a basic fault of American policy, now institutionalized through the Older Americans Act: "in the 1960's the initial policy of treating the aged as a homogeneous category was established. All aged were lumped together as a general social class with little specificity as to whether they were disadvantaged or how class, race, sex, or ethnic differences affected their status" (Estes, 1979:21). In "the aging enterprise" created by the Act, "the aged are often processed and treated as a commodity" (p. 2), thus contributing to the segregation, depersonalization, and stigmatization of the aged that the policy was supposed to overcome. Estes succumbs here and elsewhere to the categorial imperative she criticizes, for example, when talking of "a national policy that will improve life for the aged" (p. 30) and "alter the objective conditions of the aged" (p. 247). Since, however, the imperative derives in her case from the discursive dynamics of gerontology (to be discussed in subsequent chapters), rather than those of liberal humanism, her difficulty in escaping the hold of the category is only, at best, circumstantial evidence for a *cultural* coding problem.

More directly relevant is Binstock's complaint that between the early 1930s and late 1970s, well meaning "friends of the elderly" created a public rhetoric of compassionate stereotypes to combat negative ones but only, thereby, consolidated stereotypic thinking as such, providing the cognitive ground for turning the aged as a whole into a scapegoat for contemporary anxieties: "This compassionate ageism . . . set the stage for tabloid thinking about older persons by obscuring the individual and subgroup differences among them" (Binstock, 1983:140). Binstock is a liberal humanist concerned with individual differences, criticizing other humanists for being insensitive to the consequences of their public rhetoric. He would certainly endorse the comment of Wershow (1981:75) that "'*the* aged' is as pernicious a concept as are '*the* black man', '*the* oppressed female half of the world' and other counter-stereotypic stereotypes" (original emphases). Binstock too employs quotation marks to dissolve the hold of the concept, turning it into a mere label: "the current stereotypes concerning older persons are partially unwarranted and are generated by applying simplistic assumptions and aggregate statistics to a grouping called 'the aged' in order to gloss over complexities" (Binstock, 1983:140). He writes, however, as a gerontologist and could not seriously disperse one of its founding concepts without leaving the field of discourse. Consequently, we find Binstock within a few lines using "the aged" and "the old," literally, straightforwardly, and without quotation marks, to signify a single substantive entity. Binstock, like Estes, confirms in linguistic usage the integrity of a category being overtly disavowed. The coding problem of locating older persons between unique individual identity and categorial identity surfaces in gerontology as a compulsively repeated ironic figure of confirmation in denial. When Connidis (1987), having criticized positive as well as negative stereotyping, approvingly quotes a woman of 71 as saying "I don't like to be classed as a senior citizen—a part of a group. I feel I'm an individual" (p. 468), she can make of this denial of categorial identity only support for the argument that the complexity of the category needs to be respected. There is diversity among old people having "direct policy implications concerning service provision for the elderly" (Connidis, 1987:462). The individual is absorbed into a properly targeted client group for the sake of humanitarian care.

   3. *Semiotic Structure and Cultural Coding Problems.*   A. J. Greimas, applying semiotics to questions of the human production and transformation of meaning, has claimed the existence "beyond the realm of binarity, of a more complex elemental structure of signification" (cited in Schleifer, 1987:25). It is elemental in the sense of universally informing all articulations of meaning. It is complex in that the absolute minimum number of significatory units composing a meaning space is four; not one (as assumed, for example, in core value analysis) or two (as assumed in dual value analysis). The most elementary possible structure of meaning is, therefore, quadrangular, as shown in Figure 1.

A. STANDARD VERSION

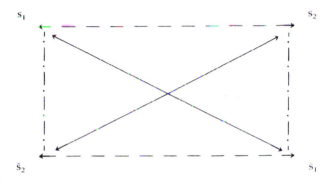

B. ALTERNATE VERSION

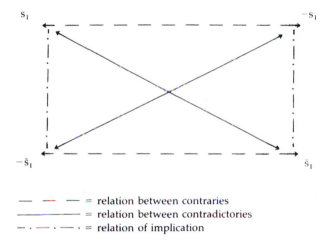

— — — = relation between contraries
————— = relation between contradictories
— · — · — · = relation of implication

Figure 1. The semiotic square of signification. *Sources:* Version A is adapted
from Schleifer (1987:25) and Greimas (1987). Version B is based on Jameson
(1972:163).

Greimas's model makes use of the traditional logical distinction between two kinds of disjunction: the active *contrary* of an idea (a positive
opposite), and a simple, passive *contradictory* (the absence of the idea). In
semantic fields, semes rather than ideas are the compositional units (in
our analysis the semes of interest being ordinary language words
worked into the discourse of gerontology), but the same kinds of rela-

tions hold good. For example, the contrary of "young" (in our culture) is "old," but its contradictory is nonyoung. The articulation of a definite seme (s_1) will then evoke a contrary definite seme (s_2), which may alternatively be designated ($-s_1$), and a contradictory negative ($\bar{s}_1$). In addition, since (s_2) is also a seme with a definite reference, it too will evoke a contradictory negative ($\bar{s}_2$), in our example, nonold.

I have given two versions of the semiotic square in Figure 1 because whereas the commonly used version (A) is useful for stressing the hierarchical relation between the top axis (signification by presence) and the bottom axis (signification by absence), where the implicatory relation between definite presence and indefinite absence is an immanent source of ambiguity, the alternative version (B) draws special attention to the problematic nature of the fourth corner of the square. In this version it is a double negative, a combination of disjunctions ($-\bar{s}_1$), dubiously related to the originary seme (s_1). Jameson (1987:xvi) refers to the "peculiar nature of the fourth term," which, in being the negation of a negation, is, therefore, a "place of novelty and of paradoxical emergence . . . the most critical position and the one that remains open or empty for the longest time" in semantic operations of the square. Where, for example, (s_1) = "the young" and ($-s_1$) = "the old," then ($-\bar{s}_1$) = the nonold who are not young yet in a relation of implication to the young. In this meaning place I would include the fabled ageless aged of far-flung Shangri-Las such as Kashmir, Georgia, and Ecuador chronicled by Dr. Leaf (Wershow, 1981:24–26), and the heroic, time-denying aged celebrated by the popular press: the senior citizen using youthful combat training to disarm a young thief, the 75-year-old marathon runner, the 68-year-old college student, and arm-wrestling "super seniors" (*Toronto Sun*, 1987:43).

We have seen that there are two immanent sources of coding difficulties built into the very structure of the semiotic square: the indefinite implications of having signs of presence underwritten by correlative signs of absence and the inherent ambiguity of double negation characterizing the fourth corner. Two further sources of coding difficulties depend on how the content of the square is specified, being, therefore, contingent rather than immanent sources but nonetheless important for that. The first is implied in Jameson's advice to analysts that in applying the square to cultural contents the four terms marking the corners "need to be conceived polysemically, each one carrying within it its own range of synonyms, and of the synonyms of its synonyms—none of them exactly coterminous with each other, such that large areas of relatively new or at least skewed conceptuality are thereby registered" (Jameson, 1987:xv–xvi). The force of the advice derives from the conviction that polysemic extension is a normal feature of all, including, analytic language practices. It belongs to the basic renaming operation of language called metonymy. The multiplication of synonyms around a primary term (for example, "the old"), in returning to complicate the equations and exchanges of an operative square becomes a source of coding problems. As Jameson suggests, the semiotic square enables us to see how metonymy, a normal operation of language, can disturb as well as confirm meaning.

Finally, the distribution of equations, differences, and exchanges in a semiotic square is greatly affected by the order of the first and second terms: "it makes a fundamental difference, in other words, whether the founding binary is ordered as white versus black, or as black versus white" (Jameson, 1987:xv). This can be seen by comparing the semantic situation of middle-aged people in an old–young versus a young–old ordering of s_1 and s_2:

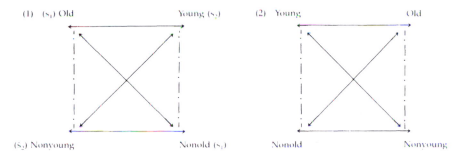

(1) (s_1) Old   Young (s_2) (2) Young   Old

$(\bar{s}_2)$ Nonyoung   Nonold $(\bar{s}_1)$ Nonold   Nonyoung

Let us say that middle-aged adults are in the third position ($\bar{s}_1$) in both cases, since it would be hard to imagine them in the nebulous fourth corner. In the first situation, their salient recognitional characteristics would be lacks and absences of being old; in the second situation they would be lacks and absences of being young. Also, in the first situation the middle-aged would be implicatively related to the young, and in the second situation, to the old.

The comparison can be sharpened by introducing a restrictive condition into the model. I would say that where cultural values are concerned, the first position (s_1) is always a positively evaluated meaning space, that is, a core value or a proxy for one, defining social desireability. We can now see the comparison in terms of the historical reversal of values described by Fischer (1978) during the nineteenth century: the switch from exaltation of age (gerontocratia) to the cult of youth (to gerontophobia). In the gerontocratic situation, the lacks and absences of the nonold would be lacks of the positive marks of the old: property, power, and established position. Moreover, implication with the young would be a threatening stigmatization to be guarded against by conspicuous distancing. In the gerontophobic situation, the semantic economy is very different. Here, the lacks and absences belonging to the position occupied by middle-aged adults are deficits in youthful characteristics: health, physical vigor, visual appeal, and openness to the future. Now it is implication with the old that has to be guarded against by conspicuous distancing. "I am not old" becomes the important message to convey, instead of "I am not young." Fitness and appearance become middle-age obsessions, while loss of openness to the future brings into social existence novel maladies such as mid-life crisis and male menopause. A rotund male stomach, once a sign of mature prosperity to be displayed in a fitted waistcoat and adorned with a watch chain, becomes a stigmatic corpulence to be hidden, dieted, or jogged away.

Being young, middle-age, or old, then, is not merely a chronological attribute, or a sociological, psychological, and biological determination, it is also a location in semiotically structured meaning spaces. In particular, meanings are organized around the semiotic square and its structurally contained ambiguities. Negotiating the square is a latent problem variously realized in every articulation of meaning. Although not the only source of cultural coding difficulties—they arise also, as we have seen, from the unacceptable marginalizing effects of accepted core values, and from value conflict—it is an abiding source that needs explicit attention in all instances of difficulty. Instances relating to old age include independence, activity, and strength. Since independence and activity are treated in subsequent chapters, I will limit discussion here to the problematic meaning of strength in relation to old age.

A term used over and again in gerontology—and for no apparent scientific reason—is frailty. The adjective *frail* seems almost automatically added in accounts of the truly old. It may be, however, that the over-again use is not just a language habit but is symptomatic of an underlying cultural coding problem concerning the equation of frailty with aging: a difficulty in settling the term within our semantic accounting systems. One such system consists of a square whose initial term (s_1) is strength:

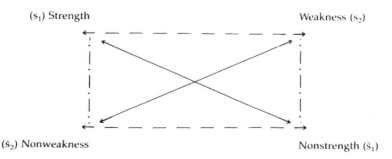

(s_1) Strength   Weakness (s_2)

($\bar{s}_2$) Nonweakness   Nonstrength ($\bar{s}_1$)

The problem is where to place frailty (and, by association, old age) in the square. At first it seems obvious that frailty belongs in (s_2), the contrary of strength, certainly if we have bodily strength in mind. Settlement is not that simple, however, since the linguistic thought of bodily weakness is culturally linked to spiritual strength, thus calling into play a semiotic square whose founding binary is spirit versus flesh, or mind versus body:

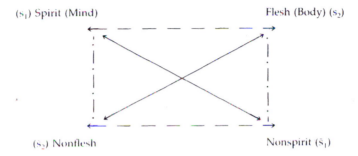

(s_1) Spirit (Mind)   Flesh (Body) (s_2)

($\bar{s}_2$) Nonflesh   Nonspirit ($\bar{s}_1$)

The second square is not transparently fastened to the first but shiftingly underlies it. We think of strong wills in weak, disabled bodies and artistic talents strongly blazing in the physically frail frames of conductors, pianists, painters, and the like.

Sally Gadow (1983) pursues these themes in an instructive essay on the dialectic of frailty and strength in philosophies of aging. She identifies three cultural frameworks for interpreting frailty: rationalistic logic, negative, nihilistic existentialism, and positive, affirmative existentialism.

Rationalist logic strictly divides spirit and flesh, mind and body, locating frailty in corporeal weakness, and interpreting it as an active negation of personal strength, the strength belonging to thought, will, and the subjective self: "Regarded strictly as object, part of the material world of decay, the aging body [i.e., frailty] can only destroy the dignity [i.e., strength] that consists in the self remaining at the centre of its experience, freely determining the nature of its relation with the body" (Gadow, 1983:145). In this cultural logic, frailty is a purely negative thing to be fought and resisted for the sake of inner strength: "the self repudiates the body to to escape being contaminated by its deterioration" (Gadow, 1983:145). In terms of the structure of the semiotic square, rationalist logic operates on the contrary relation between (s_1) and (s_2). It deals in definite contraries, being exclusively focused, therefore, on the axis of positive meaning at the top of the square and not dwelling on the axis of negative meaning ($\bar{s}_1$ $\bar{s}_2$) at the bottom. In terms of semantic content, it equates spirit with strength and body with weakness. Frailty is its name for the body/weakness equation: "when the body thwarts the projects of the self, erupting into conscious experience with the brute directness [i.e., contrariety] of the physical, frailty becomes thematic" (Gadow, 1983:144).

Turning to existentialism, the "unsmiling" kind abandons the axis of determinate contraries to dwell on the opposite axis of indeterminate negatives. It "eliminates all black-white distinctions, only to replace them with a grey and aimless ambiguity" (Gadow, 1983:145). In this interpretive frame, frailty is part of a "dirge of insoluble contradictions" (p. 145) signifying nonstrength, nonweakness, nonspirit, and nonflesh in a nonsensical existence.

Affirmative existentialism does not remain fixated on negation of positive meaning. It rounds the fourth corner of the semiotic square, the complex negation of negation that "escapes the negative/positive alternative," yielding a meaning space that is "fundamentally fecund and affirmative, and yet without positive reference" (Felman, 1983:141). In this framework, frailty becomes implicated with renewed strength: "Frailty, then, is not simply the antithesis of energy. It is itself an intense experience and brings with it new life" (Gadow, 1983:146). Frailty is here sublated from a physical weakness to an inner strength, becoming "one of the colors that an existence will have, and an especially strong color at that, neither black nor white, and certainly not grey" (Gadow, 1983:146). Frailty is, then, simultaneously nonstrength and strength, corporeality and spirituality, but only for a dialectical way of coding the world. For rationalist logic such a circling of the square would have to be an unthinkable absurdity. The differences described by Gadow concerning the interpretation of frailty and strength are not, therefore, merely value conflicts but deeper rooted cognitive divergences. It is these that generate the most radical cultural coding problems in a society.

SUMMARY

Taking up the question of how a new field of discourse called gerontology became possible and what impelled its foundation, two general conditions are identified as sufficient and necessary:

1.   A multiplication of diverse language about old age, aging, and the aged during the nineteenth century, a compound of medical, demographic, economic, humanitarian, and legislative ways making old age a legible phenomenon, which formed a dense linguistic groundwork, that is, a potential subject matter, for social science occupancy.

2.   A concomitant increase in ambiguity, ambivalence, and cognitive uncertainty about old age, aging, and the aged, that is, the development

of cultural coding problems with respect to a major area of social life. Cultural coding problems are difficulties and deficiencies in members' methods for reproducing a familiar social order. They introduce illegibilities into ordinarily legible phenomena, calling for extraordinary reflection on and about membership knowledge to half restore rational accountability to it. Religion, art, philosophy, and ideology have been historically important in performing this office but now, in modern society, it has come to be occupied by social science. Gerontology is then a social science enactment of metamembership knowledge responding to illegibility and opacity in members' methods for making old age an accountable, rationally recognizable phenomenon—a particular redoubling of membership knowledge that has become problematic in social practice.

Three forms of coding problems are those arising from the ethically distasteful marginalizing and stigmatizing effects on old people of core values, those arising from binary value conflict, and those arising from ambiguities inherent in the semiological structure of a core value. Semiological sources of ambiguity are identified through a model of signification, proposed by A.J. Greimas, called the semiotic square. The structural dynamics of the square provide for immanent sources of coding problems over and above contingencies of social change, value conflict, and so on. These are endemic to the ordinary and operative language practices of social life. Gerontology, because it is a social science tied closely to those language practices, depending on them for its production of reality and knowledge effects, cannot confine cultural coding problems to the plane of referential content but must duplicate them in its own articulations of content: in its descriptive protocols, its schemata, its models, and its theories. This is something to be further demonstrated in succeeding chapters.

CHAPTER

3

The Grammar of Dependence and Care in Gerontology

Of the several strands of discourse making up the groundwork of geron-tology, the one most important for giving interest to its subject matter is a humanitarian concern to improve the lives of elderly people and allevi-ate the problems, individual and social, of growing old. Central to the language of the humanitarian strand is a rhetoric of care *for* older people and *about* the aged as a group. It expresses both an ameliorative interest in the typical problems of individuals and a reformative interest in the situation of the group. The interests come together in public and private provisions of support services, and in the administration of expert care by professionals.

The rhetoric of care is not entirely homogeneous. The reformative interest in the group can take the direction of a search for rational alloca-tions of resources, digressing considerably from the ameliorative inter-est in individuals. (This was touched on in the previous chapter when discussing value conflicts and the paradox of liberal humanism.) Hetero-geneity can also be observed in the moral tone and emotional coloration of the rhetoric. This is illustrated by a review of American social work journals in the period 1970 to 1974, conducted by Cormican (1980). The theme of care (its strategies, tactics, and justifications) is keyed to three distinct views of aging, following a roughly chronological order of em-phasis in the period reviewed. In one view, care of the aged means protection of individuals beset by inexorable processes of role loss, mar-ginalization, and functional decline. Professional care compensates for mounting physical, psychological, and social deficits, it responds to a wish "to be cared for, protected and helped" (cited in Cormican, 1980:255) that must be presumed to exist even behind manifest resis-tance. A second view is more optimistic. The typical elderly person is vulnerable to economic, medical, and other problems but by and large remains an active, useful member of families, neighborhoods, and com-munities. Professional care for the elderly is not essentially different from other social work, a matter of supportive help, counseling, and

73

advice rather than protective, take-charge intervention. The third view emphasizes the individual diversity of aging and the aged. Care is now expressed in sensitivity to each person, awareness of the multiple patterns that need for help can take, appreciation of the diversity of valid life-style responses to aging, and attempts to tailor services to the personality, situation, and preferences of each client.

Variations in the rhetoric of care in gerontology are important and interesting. The purpose of the present chapter, however, is to seek rules of discourse operating within and below the variable play of language on the surface of the field. A useful way to formulate the problem is in terms of the transformation of ordinary language knowledge into discipline knowledge. In the everyday lifeworld, care (in the sense of caring for and caring about) is familiarly embedded in personal relationships of kinship, friendship, and love. In gerontology, care (refined now to a linguistic sign with objective references) is transferred from lifeworld contexts to scientific and professional contexts of meaning by certain operations of writing.

The problem can be posed as follows: What is done and under what rules and regularities of discourse to represent care for the elderly in gerontology? The question can be specified further by recalling the nature of the field, the fact that it is jointly oriented to human science, policy science, and moral or ethical science: to cognitive rationality, instrumental rationality, and value rationality, respectively. We can ask, then, how, in gerontological writing, care for the elderly is made legibly rational under the joint demands of scientific, instrumental, and value rationality. The question is, as implied above, basic to understanding how aging and the aged are rendered legibly rational in gerontology. The key to answering these questions is, I will argue, a circuit of discourse connecting the vocabulary of care to the vocabulary of dependence. First, however, I must present some terms of analysis.

GRAMMAR AND DISCOURSE

I have proposed that humanitarian concern for the elderly enters the field of gerontology as a circuit of discourse between two lexical clusters: one centred on the term care and the other on dependence. I would add, for subsequent reference, that although both parts of the circuit contribute to the achievement of cognitive, instrumental, and value rationality in the reading process, "care" belongs to the idea of taking action and is, therefore, especially relevant to formulating instrumental rationality (rational treatment, intervention, administration, support, and so on). "Dependence" is an identifying feature of a knowledge object, the elderly, and open to specification by formal and operational definitions. It is, therefore, especially relevant for achieving cognitive rationality (methodical description, analysis, and explanation), in the writing of gerontology. The discursive circuit from "care" to "dependence" thus contributes to that disciplinary processing of societal language materials that is the readable mark of a social science. Comparably, the return of discourse from "dependence" to "care" enacts an instrumental rationality belonging to what is called, within the field, applied gerontology.

By a circuit of discourse, I mean a patterned deployment of terms, regular ways of inserting and using them, to perform descriptions, analyses, diagnoses, predictions, strategic assessments, tactical advice, and other discursive language games. I have deliberately inserted the Wittgensteinian term, language games, because I wish to employ his concept of the grammar of language games to explore the care–dependence circuit.

Wittgenstein's concept of grammar was discussed in Chapter 1. I would like to repeat and elaborate some points made there. The most important is that analysis of the grammar underlying actual use of a word (a word, that is, with referential meaning) reveals the kind of object effected through the use: "an object-constitution is undertaken simultaneously with the drawing up of the rules of the linguistic sign. The rules of the language-game, its grammar, simultaneously determines both the use of the linguistic sign and the essential features of the object" (Specht, 1969:184). Grammatical analysis of the rules structuring the use of "care" and "dependence" in relation to "aging," "the elderly," and "the aged" should reveal, then, what these rendered objects are and can come to within the significatory system of gerontology.

Some methodological precautions are called for here. Specht refers to "the drawing up" of grammatical rules, as though they might be designed in advance of usage and operate above it, like constitutional, legal, official, and other normative prescriptions. This is not the case. The rules are *in*scribed, not *pre*scribed:

> One learns the game by watching how others play . . . we say that it is played according to such-and-such rules because an observer can read these rules off from the practice of the game—like a natural law governing the play. (Wittgenstein, 1976:Para 54)

Grammatical rules are "as if" rules reconstructed from language practices. A close model is offered by ethnomethodological reconstructions of "as if" rules in telephone transcripts and other conversational materials. When, for example, Sacks (1974) describes the accountable order of stories told by children in terms of "the economy rule," "the consistency rule," "hearer's maxims," "the sequencing rule," and "the chaining rule," he is not supposing that children or their auditors can or need to refer to the rules in so many words, only that they proceed as if they knew them. The rules are inscribed in patterns of usage. A grammar of discourse refers to textual counterparts of such rules in patterns of writing.

A grammatical proposition is "a description of the use of a sign" (Wittgenstein, 1976:Para 496), where the use has, within local bounds of discourse, the force of a necessity—a necessity, that is, for recognizably appropriate, intelligible participation in a field of discourse. Description of usage is then the basis of grammatical analysis. Achievement of description, however, is by no means straightforward. It cannot be done, for example, by treating words as representations of the objects and events they refer to, that is, describing the usage as a description of reality, because the grammar of usage precedes and makes possible the recognition of words as a description of reality, not the other way round. As Finch (1977:154–155) emphasizes, grammar comes before facts, it is "world-constituting" in the sense of allowing possible worlds to be named, searched, researched, and have determinate attributes. Neither can one simply collect descriptions in quotations, paraphrases, and the like, since these are only reproductions and not yet descriptions of usage. Following the example of ethnomethodology, what is needed is a conceptual apparatus through which to refract and formally reconstruct the rules of meaning implicit in what is being done with particular words and in what those words do in use. In a general sense, the entire vocabulary of constitutive realism, the framework of the present study, serves this purpose. For a more specific descriptive device, however, I will rely further on Greimas's semiotic model of meaning: the semiotic square (see Figure 1, in Chapter 2).

TOWARD A GRAMMATICAL DESCRIPTION OF (IN)DEPENDENCE

To provide a theme for the remainder of the chapter, I will quote what I take to be a grammatical observation by a pseudonymous author: "Kindness does not wait for an answer; care waits to be answered by dependency" (Otiosus, 1988:7).

I will first expand the second half of the aphorism. Thoughts, feelings, words, and deeds of care need to be answered by dependency in order to achieve clear meaning. Conversely, receipt of care—especially pure, unsolicited, unilateral care—confers dependency on the recipient. Benevolent purposes and sincere motives do not alter these equations, explaining both the typical resistance of old people to extensions of care and the puzzled irritation of those wanting to give care at what looks like sheer obstinacy and ingratitude. In gerontology, a regularly shaped vocabulary and syntax of dependency is interwoven with a rhetoric of care, completing a circuit of discourse in which being and becoming old are made legibly clear objects of research, ameliorative planning, and normative appraisal. Statements about being and becoming old are produced as if in conformity with necessary rules of usage. The rules can be described (or, at least, a beginning to the task can be made) through the structural dynamics and possibilities of meaning, including structured ambiguity, of a semiotic square encompassing the term independence:

(s_1) Independence   Dependence (s_2)

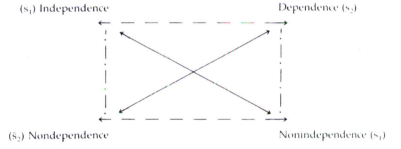

($\bar{s}_2$) Nondependence   Nonindependence ($\bar{s}_1$)

The upper axis (s_1 s_2) is the founding binary of the square. It is the axis of determinate presence, the axis of positive manifestation, where aging and the aged are made evident for theoretical and working knowledge; that is, rendered legibly real for cognitive and practical appropriation. The field requirement of being seen to do science dictates a primary orientation to the upper axis. The minimal operation here is to propose valid, reliable signs of independence and dependence so that they can be used to take the measure of old age in individuals and in populations. Dichotomous classification, however, is only the crudest form of measurement; the scientific trajectory continues by refining s_1 and s_2 into a continuum. Apart from introducing the objectifying effects of quantification, this also allows the disruptive potentiality of the lower axis ($\bar{s}_1$ $\bar{s}_2$), the axis of indeterminate negation, to be counteracted. The axis is potentially disruptive because it projects meanings parallel to concepts of (in)dependence, yet formed by negation of them, by what they are not, thus being placed outside the positive grasp of the concepts and, as in any semantic square, at the limits of scientific and instrumental cognition. Counteraction occurs through incorporating nonindependence ($\bar{s}_1$) into the s_1 s_2 continuum as a positively conceived intermediate zone. The third corner is thus absorbed into the axis of the scientific study of aging, and of rational planning to halt, ease, or reverse changes from independence to dependence.

THE CONTINUA OF CARE AND DEPENDENCY

Harris's *Dictionary of Gerontology* has the following entry under "continuum of care": "The full range of preventive, supportive, rehabilitative, and social services available in a community to older persons at various levels of need and impairments" (Harris, 1988:42). "Levels of need and impairments" refers to gradations of dependency. Specification of these renders aging a scientifically graspable phenomenon; it also provides a basis for planning arrangements for care of the aged. Recognizably rational discourse is thus doubly achieved.

Cantor and Little (1985) begin a review of social care for the elderly with a dichotomy between formal and informal care. This is called an "artificial" delimitation in the sense of being too simple to map reality. The dichotomy of care needs to be refined into continuous variables capable of being combined into an optimal mix and "proper balance" (p. 746):

> Thus the support system of the elderly can be viewed as an amalgam of kin, friends and neighbors, and societal services, each having different roles and differing relative importance at various phases in *the dependency continuum of old age*. (Cantor and Little, 1985:746–747 emphasis added)

The dependency continuum is then related back to the "spectrum of helping" existing between formal and informal kinds of care. In terms of knowledge production, the important point is not simply that the support system can be viewed as a dependency continuum, but that the continuum is an effective device through which old age can be brought to the mind's eye and held there as a determinate object for further statement. Cantor and Little offer a schematic model of the system in the graphic form of five concentric circles surrounding a central circle labeled "elderly," the circles extending from inner, closer, more personal care givers (kin; friends and neighbors), through "mediating support elements" (mailmen, shopkeepers, building superintendents, etc.), to voluntary and governmental agencies and, at the outer boundary, political and economic institutions. Supplementary distinctions represented in the model are between "nontechnical" and specialized (professional, expert) care (Cantor and Little, 1985:749), and the social scientific distinction between macro and micro levels of reality (p. 748).

The idea of nonindependence ($\bar{s}_1$ in the semiotic square) can now be determinately located along a continuum made up of overlapping dimensions. Bond (1976:13) is representative in using the concept of dependency to "synthesize the inability of an individual to carry out for him or herself the activities necessary to maintain a normative standard of everyday living." Drawing on previous studies and a panel of care professionals, he suggests five dimensions for measurement: mobility, personal self-care, housecare capacity, social isolation, and mental capacity (memory disorders, for example, are important criteria of dependency on this dimension). The first three dimensions refer to functional capacity, an especially important component of dependency in old people, and are measured through methodically sorted and ranked scale items to do with mundane activities such as climbing stairs, using public transport, bathing, cutting toenails, using the washroom, cooking, and cleaning. Paillat (1976) similarly formalizes cultural notions of an independent life and everyday knowledge of normal activities into a multiple measure of independence, showing how scales of mobility, use of free time, level of regular income, activities (i.e., incidence of freely chosen activities without pressure of need), and social contacts can be combined into an overall measure ranging from total dependence (0) to full independence (20). As he observes, a validated scale would help administrators "count 'independent' and 'dependent' old people and evaluate the efficiency of efforts made to protect this independence" (Paillat, 1976:35). On the side of scientific rationality, it would allow gerontologists to measure "transition flows from independent states to dependent ones and probabilities of transition according to various variables" (Paillat, 1976:35).

Rationality is displayed in gerontological writing not only in turning dichotomies into continua, but in making measured placement along them an expression of functional knowledge (knowledge of the differential functioning of individuals in various situations under variable conditions) rather than an exercize of taxonomic knowledge (knowledge of classificatory marks). As described in Chapter 2, Foucault (1970) associates taxonomic knowledge production with a now bygone way of recognizing the rational sense of things. In gerontology, there is a corresponding association of strong nominal classification with outdated, inappropriate, and arbitrary approaches to aging and the elderly: "In the not too distant past there was a marked division between the community and institutions for the elderly. Elderly men and women continued to live in the community as long as they were able to be independent. [If not] the only solution was institutional care, a move which often involved, and may still involve, a final and complete separation from their community" (Forbes et al., 1987:47). Rationality cannot now be seen in marked divisions but only in finely calibrated provisions of care matching constantly monitored functional wants of independence: "the often-mentioned 'continuum of care' should not only ease progression from one level of care to the next, but also a change to a different type of service, or a reduction in the level of care needed" (Forbes et al., 1987:47).

For the elderly who are between the extremes of the continuum (the nonindependent who are not fully dependent), there are "noninstitutional services": day care, vacation care, foot care, home care, nursing care, etc. Functional monitoring along the continuum is undertaken by health and welfare professionals. Increasingly, they are working in teams and units, using trained home-help aides and other caregivers as liaisons, so that care can be keyed to individually assessed dependency.

Legible rationality in giving care means a judicious inscription of individual cases along a continuum defined by objectively valid criteria of dependency: that is, an authoritative inscription. Canadian provinces, for example, have official definitions of levels of care for those in institutions (the far end of the dependency continuum). In Manitoba there are four levels of care, defined in terms of the amount of dependence an individual has on nursing time for given categories of activity: bathing, dressing, feeding, ambulation, elimination, medication, therapeutic treatment, and so on. Level 1 individuals have "minimal dependence on nursing time" for all activities; level 2 individuals have "moderate dependence" for at least one activity in a designated subset; level 3 individuals have "maximum dependence" for two or three categories in a designated subset; and level 4 individuals have maximum dependence for four or more categories (Forbes et al., 1987:19). British Columbia has a five level schema, also based on time rationing for categories of care, but more finely calibrated. "Personal care" requires no individual attention, only general, nonprofessional supervision; "Intermediate care 1 (IC-1)" requires up to 75 minutes of individual attention per day, 15 minutes professional and 60 minutes nonprofessional; "Intermediate care 2 (IC-2)" calls for 100 minutes attention in the ratio of 30 professional and 70 nonprofessional minutes; "Intermediate care 3 (IC-3)" calls for 120 minutes in the ratio of 30 professional and 90 nonprofessional minutes; "Extended care" means round the clock professional supervision and at least 150 minutes of individual attention per day, most of it through a "multi-disciplinary therapeutic team" (Forbes et al., 1987:20).

I take it that continuous measurement and monitoring of dependency underlie provisions for old age in all modern jurisdictions, and throughout the (in)dependence continuum of care. One can see the pattern of usage again, for example, in public and private housing arrangements for the elderly. A review of housing options in Ontario, Canada (*Toronto Life*, 1988) includes, in order of dependency level: nursing homes (at least 75% of beds must be for extended care, i.e., 90 minutes of nursing care per day, directed by a doctor), homes for the aged (offering both extended care, as above, and "residential care," i.e., less than 90 minutes nursing and individual attention per day), retirement homes (limited nursing and personal care but with professional medical care on call), seniors' apartments, "granny flats," "Abbeyfield houses" (group homes for 7 to 10 residents plus a housekeeper, designed to allow seniors with minor functional incapacities to stay in their local neighborhoods), retirement villages, and seniors' co-ops (run by resident-owners and designed for "independent living"). Private households are primarily locales of independence but home care support services allow for continuous gradations of "supported independent living" (Novak, 1988:223). Retirement villages and the like are internally structured by the same rule of rationality. In the United States, Life Care Communities offer self-contained units for independent living, supplemented by a complete range of medical, therapeutic, and personal care services. A report on an experimental retirement community in Coventry, England, says: "Residents will be able to move through the various degrees of housing or nursing care *in situ*, remaining close to their friends and neighbors" (*The Sunday Telegraph*, 1988).

It is my argument that whatever disagreements exist about the particulars of old age policy, there is an implicit agreement about the meaning of a rational provision of care: a shared way of recognizing it. Moreover, this agreement runs through the field of gerontology as well as social administration, being part of a grammatical contract of discourse about care. In the contract is a rule that the term care can and, for maximum rational effect, should be mapped onto a measurable continuum running from independence to dependence. Its grammar of usage dictates that care is a measurable and distributable kind of thing. It can and should be spoken of in the way of all such things—in, for example, the language of supply and demand, cost–benefit analysis, and delivery systems. I will return to Cantor and Little (1985) for illustration.

To address the question of how well the needs of older Americans are being met, they ask, in completely conventional fashion: "how does the system operate to provide the necessary assistance?" (Cantor and Little, 1985:747). Following a distinction between informal and formal subsystems, "the delivery of formal services" is criticized for lack of systematicity:

> Ideally, a social service delivery system translates resources into assistance. Unfortunately, fragmented policy over time has created not one but several service systems in the United States, making for considerable fragmentation and sometimes duplication of effort. (Cantor and Little, 1985:767)

The regulative ideal of systems rationality, exactly matching the distribution of care along a continuum of dependency, makes fragmentation of care a self-evident fault, and duplication even worse. Provision of assistance in the United States (and Canada) lacks legible rationality because "there is no single entry point into a single service delivery system" (p. 768). The Scandinavian and British welfare state systems are places of superior care because they have a "comprehensive, integrated, personal social service system with a delivery outlet in each locality" (p. 769). They are places (places, that is, in gerontological discourse) where care can be "seen" graphically as a measured entirety and thus rendered in writing a rational phenomenon. (What these places might be "in reality," beyond discourse, is another question—probably metaphysical—that I will not take up.) The point I want to stress, and take a little further, is that the continuum of care is not simply a response to prior needs of the old, it is, in conjunction with the dependency continuum, a means of making the old a determinate knowledge object.

THE COGNITIVE FUNCTION OF THE CARE–DEPENDENCY CONTINUUM

Georg Simmel's classical essay on the poor as a social category ends with what I take to be a grammatical statement (in Wittgenstein's sense) about the constitution of the category:

> Thus, what makes one poor is not the lack of means. The poor person, sociologically speaking, is the individual who receives assistance because of this lack of means. (Simmel, 1971:178)

Giving assistance in money or kind makes needy individuals socially recognizable—hence, describable, classifiable, and legibly knowable— as the poor. It can be asked, then, through what kind of social act elderly individuals are, in our form of society, made known as the old. The answer I am advancing is that the category is constituted in acts of care correspondent to dependency. The old, like the poor, is a social category formed by what is done *to* and *for* its members rather than by what they do. To be one of the old is to be in a passively defined meaning space. This is why active individuals old in years are figures of cultural curiousity and interest, capable, for example, of sustaining dramatic plots and human interest media stories. It is also why the most definitely formed, firmly known, and legibly clear old people are those on whom the most frequent and various acts of care-for-dependency are performed: those called in gerontology the old–old or the frail elderly—*the* old in very deed. Whatever their numerical, or other "real world" importance they provide gerontology with a relatively stable reference point and reliable anchorage of meaning. This is one reason why "the frail elderly" has become, through repeated use, something like a technical term in the field. Harris's *Dictionary of Gerontology* defines it as follows: "Older persons with mental, physical, and/or emotional disabilities that limit their independence and necessitate continuing assistance; persons 75 years or older" (Harris, 1988:75). The definition begins to indicate the variety of meanings attached to the term dependency in the lexicon of the field. I will examine the variety of use more closely in order to detail the connection of compound dependency to cognitive clarity.

Drawing on Harris once more, her definition of dependence includes reliance on others for "physical, economic, mental and/or social supports" (Harris, 1988:52). The four subcategories of dependency listed here separately underlie other social prototypes: the physically disabled, the poor, the mentally disabled, and the isolated. In the truly old they are synthesized into a single category correlated with being over a certain age. [Harris says 75 years but Havens (1980), using statistical analysis to find the cutting point at which needs for physical, medical, economic, and social supports decisively accumulate, says age 80 for males and 85 for females.]

The exact age marker is subject to change, as is the verbal label of the category. The particular labels in current circulation, the "old–old" and "frail elderly," are only contingencies of discourse on aging and the aged, but the formation of a compound dependency category for marking and labeling is a grammatical necessity. When, for example, Marshall (1987:477) calls the distinction between the "old–old" and "young–old" a "ridiculous," "cavalier" usage, and satirizes the term "frail elderly" as a "new buzz word" in the professional vocabulary, he is only tilting at contingent windmills. The care–dependency circuit giving sense and discursive exchange value to the terms Marshall ridicules is essential to the field in which he is making utterances. Consequently, he can rhetorically reject the terms but not escape the grammar of usage they represent. Even though it is "obviously ridiculous to talk about 'the aged'" (p. 477) and classify the aged into the old–old and young–old, Marshall's announced topic refers to the "health of the very old people," and they are then located demographically within "the aged group" (p. 474). The group is made substantially recognizable and further specifiable in terms of measurable needs across a broad spectrum of dependency. Marshall is then able to talk unridiculously about delivering services to "the elderly" (p. 477) and "public policies for the support of the aged" (p. 483). The fault of the old–old, young–old distinction it turns out is not in being made but in being insufficiently rigorous to specify dependency needs and care delivery. When specification is done, cognitive clarity is restored to "the aged" and the term can be used again straightforwardly, without hesitation marks. The point I would emphasize is that the specification is grammatically pegged to a multiple concept of dependence fashioned scientifically from culturally known want of independence. Scientific fashioning includes, above all, measurement. Categories of dependence can be thought of then as coordinates intersecting variously in individuals and sets of individuals. The greater the number of dependency coordinates combined in an individual, the more legibly definite the individual is as an old person.

Further to the multiple meanings of dependency, the four categories (or coordinates) in Harris's definition need to be expanded to include demographic and psychological dependency. The latter is anticipated in the inclusion of emotional disability in the definition of the frail elderly given previously. Munnichs (1976:5) formally distinguishes instrumental from individual (in)dependence, the first term relating to everyday activities and functional competence, and the second to "the 'autonomy' of the personality." Lack of autonomy in chronically dependent personalities is distinguished from temporary "crisis dependency" and normal developmental (transition) dependency. It is a pathological "neurotic dependency" expressed in "self-effacement, dread of loneliness, ingratiation and indecision" (p. 5). Cantor and Little make a similar distinction between normally developing instrumental dependency and pathological inner dependency: "as persons grow older and frailer most societies look with greater tolerance on their needs for assistance and support. Dependency in these contexts is normal, not pathological" (Cantor and Little, 1985:746).

Normal dependency, then, is correspondent with objectively needed and socially approved care for the common infirmities of old age, while pathological dependency is correspondent with a compulsive, subjective need for dependence itself. Of course, the task of distinguishing one from the other, thus separating care for the functionally frail from therapy for the inwardly disabled, and the clearly old from the psychologically ill, is most delicate. Some attributes of frailty, like emotional disability and social isolation, have the same recognitional signs as neurotic dependency. Moreover, the behaviors might arise from social location rather than a disordered personality system. Ujimoto (1987:117) points out that many aged immigrants are linguistically and culturally cut off from social means of expressing feeling, obtaining mutual recognition, and asserting oneself, thus posing problems of interpreting their behavior. Clearly, the identification of psychological dependency in old people demands expert knowledge of personality systems and the inner functioning of individuals.

Does psychological dependency belong to the definition of being old, to the care–dependency continuum along which that category is produced and made recognizable, or is it only a hazard, a contingency, of becoming old? As a medical syndrome in psychiatry, psychological dependency is not a defining feature of being old. However, as a connotation (being childish, unreasonably demanding, unable to care for oneself, and so on) in the linguistic means for recognizing old age, it belongs with the other meanings of dependency in the cognitive composition of the aged. It colors the entire meaning space in which the aged is made a legible object.

There remains one other component of the spectrum of dependency, that provided by demography. The key concept here is the age dependency ratio. Technically, this is the ratio of the number of persons under 15 and over 65 years of age in a population to the number aged 15–64. However, the connotations that make it reasonable for those under 15 and over 65 to be added together as the dependent population are economic, interactional, and psychological. The concept is, therefore, discursively integrated with the rest of the spectrum. As will be explained in the next chapter, this is of the utmost importance in allowing demography to give topical coherence to a multidisciplinary field. Meanwhile, I wish only to illustrate the scope of the concept across the spectrum of dependence.

Monk (1980) employs the concept to discuss the economics of aging and the social, political, and ethical problems of transferring funds from a present working generation to one that has ceased to work, especially where transfers are also intended to be large enough to shelter the old from poverty. The dependent population is equated with "the nonproductive segment of our economy" (Monk, 1980:42), and the concern raised by the age dependency ratio is "how many productive people it takes to support a nonproductive older person" (p. 44).

I should add that Monk is critical of negative sentiments fomented by the rising old-age dependency ratio. Like other critics, however, he misconstrues the problem of dependency and old age, treating it as a matter of feelings and attitudes rather than one of reality construction and how the old are made known. Dependency is, for Monk, as for any substantive realist, something *in* a prior object (here, the old) that then, like a sensory attribute, stimulates responses. The position I take, that of constitutive realism, locates dependency in our methods for producing a knowledge object and making old age real, legible and cognitively evident. Methods that include the unremarkable transfer of dependency from the assembly process to the assembled object as *its* attribute, thus achieving constitutive innocence for the act of cognition and object-like facticity for its product.

Our responses to the growing ratio of nonproductive, dependent elderly are, Monk complains, irrational. By which he means that they are disproportionate and faulty. However, resentment, hostility, and other expressions of stigmatic marginalization are perfectly consistent with dependency, being indeed, as was shown in the previous chapter, dictated by its logic. The responses referred to by Monk are, therefore, at least value rational. The fault, if fault there be, is in the way we are rational, not in our being irrational. Warnings against equating old age with dependency and thus visiting on elderly people the unhappiness of a stigmatic label are helpless against the epistemological fact that it is through the concept of dependence that old age comes into social existence. When Estes (1979:5) makes it a matter of remediable complaint that "the aged are perceived as dependent," she misses the point that dependency is the cognitive matrix through which "the aged" takes determinate form and has definite existence. Exhortations to dissolve the age–dependency equation and remove the label from the category are impossible requests to think an object while dispensing with the indispensable means of thinking it.

What can be done, and what gerontology does to inscribe scientific and instrumental rationality in its subject matter, is to refine the concept of dependency. Instead, therefore, of simply equating demographically defined dependency with financial, physical, societal, and personal dependency, gerontologists calculate age-related probabilities of falling into differential types and degrees of dependence. Regarding health care, for example, where individual signs of functional and financial dependency intersect with budgetary calculations of aggregate burden, it is emphasized that "while the elderly as a group use large amounts of medical services, the pattern is not uniform across this population segment" (Montgomery et al., 1987:237). A demographically based attempt to include the pattern in measures of population aging can be seen in the disability-free life expectancy index proposed by Wilkins and Adams (1983). For any population group, the expected years of long-term institutionalization and disability are subtracted from life expectancy in the group: "this sophisticated index allows an examination of how the later years of life differ from one group to another. It permits some degree of insight into the real economic burdens placed on certain subgroups of society" (McDaniel, 1986:14). It also promotes a more finely knit discursive integration of the dependency spectrum and thus a more assured cognitive grasp of aging and the aged.

The same dynamic, binding integration of the dependency spectrum to the cognitive legibility of the aged appears on the *applied* front of dependency: the *provision* of care. For example, the marked and repeated concern of American gerontologists with the multiplicity of provisions for care and points of entry in their system (or as some say, satirically, their nonsystem) is not immediately understandable. Why is it "a major weakness of the U.S. non-system" to lack "a universal gateway or doorway to service"? (Cantor and Little, 1985:771). Is it not a major strength of the American polity to give citizens plural access to the public sphere and multiple gateways to service? And if "the older American is faced with many private providers who may or may not be known to the individual and may or may not relate to each other," is this not the ideal situation of the free market consumer, and the best guarantee of efficiency and satisfaction? Short of attributing to gerontologists either a subversive, anti-American collectivism or unthinking system fetishism, it is hard to understand their need to see inscribed in the provisions for care "the three C's: comprehensiveness, continuity, and coordination" (cited in Cantor and Little, 1985:771). My proposal, touching a theme that will be variously expounded here and in subsequent chapters, is that the need is epistemological rather than ideological. Comprehensiveness, continuity, and coordination need to be seen (i.e., to be legibly present) in provisions for care so as to certify the same features in its conceptual correlate, the dependency continuum, this being, in turn, the discursive ground for rendering old age a coherent knowledge object (i.e., an object of comprehensive, continuous, and coordinated study).

The same epistemological need is at work, I would argue, in attributing objective wants of care to elderly people regardless of their expressed wants. The old are objectified in objective dependency. I take this to be another expression of the grammar of care and dependence in gerontology.

A typical case of its operation is a Canadian research report by Cape (1987) on "one of the most hidden of all subgroups of seniors" (Cape, 1987:85): older rural females. At present they are known only "in demographic silhouette" (p. 86). Cape's task then is to endow a shadowy knowledge object with discursive substance, to draw it into the field of gerontology, and articulate the dimensions of its reality, which in this field means the dimensions of aging. Her primary articulation device, obedient to the grammar under discussion, is a demonstration that, regardless of appearances, there are unmet needs for care along the dependency spectrum. The grammar is evident in a discursive operation whereby data suggesting normal independence and no need for special provisions of care, *hence no research readable presence of aging*, are reworked to show the actual dependency and need hidden by appearances, thus revealing the real elderliness of the demographic silhouette.

Cape says that her data generally support the belief that rural communities are places of personal contact and mutual help where functional independence is commonly maintained in later years. However, it takes only a little conjecture, hypothesis, and projection to see what, grammatically, has to be seen. Not all rural elderly women are in fact rural. There is an "increasing in-migration of urban elders who may or may not have close ties to their new community" (p. 96). Only longitudinal research will establish whether the "rural roots" of city wives will have grown sufficiently strong to "cope with advancing age and widowhood" (p. 97). In any case, no matter how strong the roots "only so much can be done informally: the services of kinfolk and peers may be necessary, but they are not sufficient for meeting the dependency needs of old age and widowhood" (p. 96).

Hypothetical conjecture is again used to rework the finding that most of the elderly women interviewed said they did not need special assistance and got along perfectly well without it—being, therefore, only nominally and not researchably old. Cape speculates that the really incapacitated must be somewhere else, in special care: "Had they been more incapacitated, it is unlikely that they would have been able to remain in the community" (Cape, 1987:97), adding that the greater involvement of "visiting homemakers" with the most elderly categories is "a straw in the wind" attesting to "the rising incidence of medically defined incapacity" (p. 97). I do not say that Cape as an individual researcher is grasping at straws, but that any gerontological researcher, to work in the field, must see evidence of dependency needs calling for provisions of care. This is how gerontology turns what would otherwise be mere chronological categories into substantively full and complex objects of inquiry.

Even gerontologists sensitive to the possible harm of equating age with dependency (inadvertently reinforcing the prejudices of "ageism" that gerontology would combat) are constrained in the event, the event of field discourse, to observe the grammar of care for dependency. Connidis (1987), for instance, shows constitutive sensitivity in warning that "the type of attention paid to the subject of aging often tells more about our view of aging than it does about old age" (p. 451). Also in a constitutive vein is her observation that just as sociology has a "fundamental material interest" in seeing social problems wherever it looks, so agencies providing care to the elderly have a vested interest in seeing problems of aging. In both cases, what it is profitable to see is seen. Connidis's constitutive insight is limited, however, to the idea of selective perception shaped by external interests, it does not extend to the inner conditions of reality and knowledge production. It does not extend to the constitutive necessities of gerontology, including its grammar of care for dependency, which are not means of achieving prestige, funding, and the like, but are internal conditions for making coherent, appropriate statements in its field of discourse. Connidis proceeds to meet these conditions. Like Cape, she relies upon the care-dependency circuit to render old age a substantively full knowledge object, reworking even unpromising materials to find instantiations of it.

The circuit is activated by observing that although the negative stereo-type of total dependency is unrealistic so also is the positive stereotype of active independence promoted by champions of the elderly. [Con-nidis comes unwittingly close to a grammatical truth when she says there are those "who espouse a positive view so unrealistic that it bor-ders on denial" (1987:454). What the denial of dependence would deny, however, is the possibility of producing the knowledge object, the aged, not the reality of aging.] Between these unreal poles is the spectrum, the care–dependency continuum, where the reality of aging is to be found.

Once in play, the circuit dictates what data will count as relevant, how information will be interpreted, what kinds of questions and problems will guide research, and, in ethnographic studies, which respondents will be quoted as telling voices, and what their voices will be said to tell. Connidis, for example, quotes two women from her study of older peo-ple in London, Ontario, who expressed disinterest in activities and ser-vices for senior citizens, the second adding: "I don't like to be classed as a senior citizen—a part of a group. I feel I'm an individual" (p. 468). These women could be heard, outside gerontology, to be resisting the categorial basis of care for dependency, and challenging the validity of the grammar. Connidis, however, within the bounds of the grammar, takes them to tell of "the diversity among old people, a diversity that has direct policy implications concerning *service provision for the elderly*" (p. 462, emphasis added), thus reasserting the discursive authority of the dependency category in the act of acknowledging its diversity. Similarly, the grammar dictates that the significant thing about the finding that 90% of the elderly respondents liked the stage of life they were in, is that 10% liked nothing about it. The latter segment is made the analytic focus of attention because it is here that the truly old, replete with "the prob-lems of aging" (p. 469), can be recognized and formulated. In the gram-mar of care for dependency, unproblematic elders cannot be recognized as really, legibly old. Gerontology cannot be written about them.

COGNITIVE TENSIONS IN THE GRAMMAR
OF (IN)DEPENDENCE

Having stressed the role of the grammar of (in)dependence in making old age a legible, discursively graspable phenomenon, I should point also to cognitive tensions built into its operation. These can be traced to the fact that gerontology is constitutively formed around three kinds of rationality—scientific, instrumental, and value (or cultural) rationality—each with its own conditions of discursive accomplishment. The most strongly marked division, and the one most fraught with cognitive tension, is that between scientific and cultural rationality. There is indeed an inherent contradiction between their conditions of achievement, one that can identified through the semiotic square of independence given earlier in the chapter. For convenience, I reproduce it here, with an added specification of the labeling to suit the present discussion:

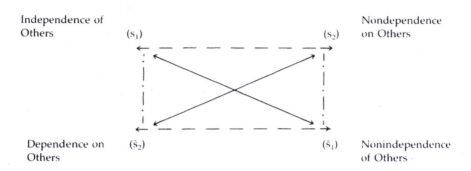

Independence of Others (s$_1$)   Nondependence on Others (s$_2$)

Dependence on Others (s̄$_2$)   Nonindependence of Others (s̄$_1$)

The square *as a whole* describes an elementary structure of meaning (individual independence) in the cultural code, the self-collective representations, of our society. The society, that is, to which the field of gerontology belongs and to whose members' methods of knowledge production it is bound. Display of cultural rationality in accounts of old age depends, therefore, on instantiating the square and reproducing its pattern of differences.

I have described the grammar of dependence in gerontology as a regulated usage rather than mere reproduction of the semiotic square. Restrictions and extensions of word use are imposed on the elementary structure of meaning to fit the requirements of scientific rationality. The rules of the revisionary grammar require: (1) confinement of usage to the positive upper axis (s$_1$ s$_2$), where conceptual definiteness and operational exactness of meaning can be sought, (2) conceptualization of the difference between independence and dependence as a divisible continuum rather than a binary opposition, (3) incorporation of nonindependence (s̄$_1$) into the positive axis as a set of intermediate values on the (s$_1$ s$_2$) continuum, and (4) treatment of any situations beyond the conceptual grasp of the continuum as beyond the scope of positive knowledge about aging. My argument is that to sustain the social intelligibility of gerontology, cultural requirements (the logic of the total semiotic square of independence) must work their way back into the scientifically oriented revision of the square—a process necessarily accompanied by cognitive stress and strain.

Two linguistic signs of cognitive stress in a discourse are conceptual paradox and conceptual strangeness. By conceptual strangeness I do not mean the estrangement of familiar topics from ordinary language through technical terms—a normal appropriation procedure of social science, to be discussed in the next chapter—but conjunctions and applications of ordinary language terms that strike an ordinary language member as strange.

Conceptual paradox appears in attempts to give the negative third corner of the square, nonindependence ($\bar{s}_1$), a positive name and thus integrate it conceptually into the (in)dependency continuum. Methodical efforts in this direction occur in a collection of papers on dependency in old age edited by Munnichs and van den Heuvel (1976). Munnichs asks in his lead-off essay: "Are there no modi between dependency and independency which reflect better the concrete situation in which many people find themselves?" (Munnichs, 1976:4). He argues for the greater realism of in-between conditions and advocates the term "interdependency" to describe them. This insertion is a seemingly innocent and sensible concession to reality but it turns out in textual practice to undermine and subvert the difference between independency and dependency that it is designed to supplement, in effect, ruining the integrity of the semiotic square and the elementary structure of value meanings it represents. An intimation of this is glimpsed in a paradoxical aside added by Munnichs to his claim of the greater correspondence of the term interdependency to reality: "For instance, even the independent person is for his work already dependent on the help that the dependent person needs" (p. 4).

The paradox of the independent person being actually dependent is expanded to almost Hegelian proportions by another contributor to the collection. Solem (1976), having defined dependency as low access to individual and/or environmental resources, reasons that where environmental resources are scarce for everyone "the independent individual has one horse to gamble on," namely oneself, consequently "the independent individual is dependent upon his own individual resources" (p. 77). Solem then generalizes his semantic exploration of nonindependence along the (in)dependency continuum into a culturally relevant commentary: "Every human being is dependent, both upon individual and environmental resources. . . . In societies leaning heavily on individual independency as a social value, the person independent of the environment is called independent. But the more independent he is of environmental resources, the more dependent he is upon his own individual resources" (pp. 77–78).

Van den Heuvel (1976), in the same collection, attributes the confusing multiplicity of meanings of dependency in the literature to lack of "a frame of reference about dependency" (p. 162). My diagnosis is somewhat different. Technical definitions of dependency can be integrated in gerontology, as we have seen, on a hypothetical continuum. These cannot, however, be integrated with ordinary language, cultural definitions of dependence and independence. The reason for this irreconcilability is semiotic. The two kinds of definition belong to different and incompatible structures of meaning.

Cultural definitions belong to the elementary structure of meaning in ordinary language: a fourfold structure of binary pairs that defines what dependency is through what it is not.

Technical definitions belong to a refined structure of meaning worked up from and against ordinary language: a bipolar continuum that defines dependency by relative amounts of positive indicators (physical, mental, emotional, financial etc.).

These two structures of meaning correspond to two frames of reference and two forms of rationality ultimately at odds with each other: on the one hand to technical knowledge and system rationality and on the other hand to everyday understanding and lifeworld rationality. It is the fate (and fortune) of every social science to be pulled between these two frames of thought at every turn, so it is futile to hope for a single frame of reference about dependency or any other topic in gerontology. Van den Heuvel is closer to the truth when he adds to lack of a frame of reference the problem of reconciling diverse frames of reference—those of scientists, policy-makers, care professionals, and the elderly themselves. He seems to imagine this, however, as an ethical and political problem of fair compromise belonging to the context of the field, rather than a cognitive problem built into the very constitution of the field itself and into its literary texture.

Conceptual strangeness, the other linguistic sign of cognitive tension generated in and by the grammar of dependence, appears in attempts to conceptually capture states of dependence so total and extreme that they seem beyond any conceivable continuum with independence—a condition virtually beyond the recognitional grasp of independency, interdependency, and dependency, yet somehow having to be positively named for the sake of scientific identification and research. In the structure of the semiotic square the condition belongs to the ever-ambiguous fourth corner ($\bar{s}_2$), a compound negation of negations of independence that is, thereby, curiously implicated with it: almost like a shadow image or inverse negative of independence. Positive science cannot grasp such meaning—it is, like every content of the fourth corner, a matter of poetry, fantasy, or metaphysics—yet *social* science is compelled to try because such meaning is integral to the elementary structures constituting social reality and social knowledge. Such attempts are inevitably marked by conceptual strangeness. An example in gerontology of attempting to grasp the fourth corner of independence is provided by the concept of social death.

Kalish (1966) locates social death along "a continuum of subjectively perceived death," calling it a condition where a person is defined or treated by others as dead even though medically alive. It is distinguished from "psychological death" where the individual defines himself or herself as being as good as dead.

The conceptual strangeness of social death, where an adjective is applied to a noun that nullifies it, is underlined in accounts of its presence in the continuum of care, the operational counterpart of the dependency continuum. Gustafson (1981), for example, drawing on Roth's study of TB patients, describes a timetabled death "career" among nursing home patients. A nursing home is, in the continuum of care, "the last resource for old people" when other resources of "social independence" have been exhausted: "Admission to a nursing home is widely considered the ultimate failure in one's social career. Roth himself perceives the nursing home patient as a 'career failure' . . . He claims that life in such a cul-de-sac is not a career because it moves in no direction" (Gustafson, 1981:505).

Roth is describing, in effect, an absolute individual, someone beyond the goals, expectations, rewards, and punishments mediated by others, therefore beyond social definition. Gustafson is not ready to give up so soon on the sociality of nursing home patients, nor to relax the hold of the grammar of dependence in describing them. She describes a "timetable of social death" (p. 205), prior to the "terminal phase," during which patients assert their social presence (including their continuing claim to be judged by the cultural criterion of independency) against consignment by others (relatives, friends, staff) to "premature social death" (p. 515). The assertion is called "a justifiable fight" and also a "kind of bargaining" to postpone social death. The terminal phase is "beyond the bargaining process," that is, beyond social life, interdependency, independency, and dependency. It is a liminal movement toward absolute independence: "Only when the patient moves into the terminal phase should he feel he is bargaining directly with God for more time" (p. 516). Only then can the individual be declared socially exorbitant, hence beyond the orbit of the grammar of dependence and beyond the grasp of social scientific discourse. Grammars of meaning scan semiotic materials incessantly and exhaustively for instantiations of their patterns, inspecting everything within interpretable range as a possible instance and recognizable replica. The fourth corner of the semiotic square of independence represents a defeat, an opacity, an illegible meaning for the grammar of independence in that it projects an idea of absolute independence, thus exceeding the socially defined idea which is the basis of the grammar.

POWER–KNOWLEDGE AND THE SYNTAX
OF DEPENDENCY

The observation made above that a grammar of usage is not just a set of rules waiting to be applied, but an active scanning device playing on semiotic materials to produce realizations of itself, recalls Foucault's thesis (discussed in Chapter 2) that knowledge, especially of human reality, is always a joint power–knowledge operation. In the present case, recognitional scanning of bodies, behaviors, activities, and inactivities for signs of dependency and needs for care draws attention to the power side of the tandem. This is most evident in instrumentally rational formulations of the aged as an object of caregiving: in designed provisions of support, aid, rehabilitation, and cure.

The concept of recognitional scanning includes both macro- and microlevel power effects. Foucault's *Discipline and Punish* can be read as a study of the different recognitional functions of penal methods in different forms of society, that is, within different means of collective self-representation. A social sovereign is made recognizable in displays of absolute power on the bodies of criminals, in public spectacles of maiming, humiliation, and death; society as civil contract is recognized in repayments, restorations, and paying debts to society; a social system, the modern form of society, recognizes itself in rehabilitative treatments to restore and optimize individual functionality within societal parameters. Assessment, monitoring, testing, and therapy are as self-evidently rational penal methods in system recognition as public torture in sovereign recognition, and the fine calculation of degrees of deprivation for classes of offense in contract recognition. The same themes of assessment, monitoring, and functional optimization are evident, as we have seen, in modern formulations of the aged. They structure the design of institutional provisions of care and are reproduced in the practical details of caregiving to ensure their rational accountability.

Michel de Certeau, following Foucault's path, has, with critical intent, examined techniques of power–knowledge, the "microbe-like operations" (Certeau, 1984:xiv) enfolding and permeating individuals in strategic locales like schools, administrative offices, and hospitals. Especially relevant is his observation that in such locales the "thinkable" (the meaningful, the significant) is identified with what can be done. In hospitals, for example, "to care for means to cure" (Certeau, 1984:190). In this context, the dying person becomes an affront to reason by becoming "an object that no longer makes itself available to be worked upon by others" (p. 190). For instrumental rationality, a dying person is a lapse of discourse, a breach of cognitive order, hence "ob-scene" (p. 191).

The recognizeably old are past work but not, until the last extreme of dependency, past being worked on. The old are "thinkable" and meaningful as long as and to the extent that they can be inscribed in the care–dependency circuit. This is why they are kept within it so thoroughly and solicitously. Caregiving is crucial for securing the rational accountability of the category and, thereby, the social order—the reproductive order of power–knowledge—to which it belongs.

Interactional scanning for dependency in professional and technocratic contexts can easily be linked to the exercize of power in the usual sense, and the gerontology literature is not lacking in awareness of or sensitivity to the matter. Dowd (1981), for example, uses a power–dependency exchange theory from political sociology to explain how the aged suffer a chronic deficit in their balance of exchange relations with others, in their relative ability to mediate goals for others, which they pay for in compliance, the standard currency of the weak. Having relatively little of exchange value to offer others means "an increased dependence upon others and the concomitant necessity to comply to their wishes" (Dowd, 1981:73). He adds that unbalanced exchange rates can easily become institutionalized and regarded as normal, as in the case of the aged.

Observations such as these are useful for describing contingencies of action but they do not address grammars of usage. When Dowd refers to a necessity of compliance, for example, he means a necessity of causal sequence, not of reality construction and knowledge production: empirical (contingent) rather than constitutive (grammatical) necessity. This is shown by the fact that Dowd entertains a political solution to the balance of dependence deficit. Another way for the aged to redress their imbalanced exchange situation, he argues from the theory, is to form coalitions with other age groups. The one major obstacle he can see to the solution is purely temporary and contingent: "the aged themselves have yet to develop any extensive awareness of their common social and economic plight, which is a necessary prerequisite to entering into coalitions" (Dowd, 1981:76). My objection to this is that the "common plight" of "the aged" is not social or economic but epistemological. What the aged have in common is subjection to certain conditions and procedures of recognition, certain methods of knowledge production, central to which is the grammar of dependence. This means that only through the grammar can someone be recognized as being old; conversely, without conforming in some degree to its definitional prescriptions, one cannot be recognizeably old. Consequently, the idea of organizing on the basis of old age to resist and reduce dependency is grammatically absurd. The wants of the aged would have to be conveyed in the vocabulary of dependency to be comprehensible and the vocabulary cannot be used without reproducing the grammar. The organization would, therefore, have to reinstate dependency in resisting it. Should such an organization, moreover, become powerful it would be seen as a group speaking *for* the aged, not as a group *of* the aged. The dependency division between care providers and care recipients would thus be reproduced within the political organization of the group.

The argument that the vocabulary of dependence (the care–dependency circuit of discourse) cannot be used without reproducing the grammar of dependency applies also, of course, to the field of gerontology. Even gerontologists critical of couching the old in terms of dependency will ineluctably reproduce the grammar of those terms. It is constitutive of any legible discourse on being and becoming old in our society, regardless of the rhetorical direction and intent of such discourse. To substantiate the argument it is helpful to consider the syntax of dependency statements.

By syntax of dependency I mean that sentences linking the aged (or the old, or the elderly) to care are structured by prepositions and verbs casting the category in a passive, dependent position. The syntax asserts, regardless of intent, an active–passive, us–them power division between reader and writer (the actants of discourse) on the one hand, and the aged (the subjects of utterance) on the other. Some illustrations will clarify the idea. They are passages taken at random from the gerontology literature. All emphases, drawing attention to the syntax, have been added.

Kreps (1966), discussing "employment policy and income maintenance *for the aged*" (p. 136), attributes slow progress to "society's failure to agree on the goals of policy *for the aged*" (p. 137), but finds encouragement in the fact that "media for publicly *transferring* income *to the aged*" are already in place (p. 152). She believes that once the aged have been guaranteed minimum incomes "the problem of *providing them* some share of the national product can be met" (p. 154). Novak (1988:181) says that a goal of the Canadian retirement income system is "to *keep all older people out of* poverty." Novak (1988:223) exhibits a chart showing a "continuum of housing by degree of independence," with a note added that "a good system *gives* people the support they need, while *allowing them* to do as much for themselves as they can." Davies (1985), discussing health care and the aged, says that the United States does not "*provide* comprehensive health care *for* all age groups" but "*targets* some special assistance *for* the aged" (p. 731). Kane and Kane (1981), discussing "*care for the aged*" (p. 477) and alternatives to institutional care, refer approvingly to the British system where "a geriatric hospital service is used to assess new admissions on a *triaging* function" (p. 478). (A triage is a sorting operation, applied especially to sorting out broken coffee beans. An assessment and monitoring service called TRIAGE is said to be operating in Connecticut.) In the British system "patients *deemed* rehabitable *for* community living are *routed into* appropriate treatment units" (p. 478). Truly it is said that "we do social welfare *to* old people and not with them" (Johnson, 1976:159, original emphasis).

To complete the argument I will cite the case of a gerontologist speaking against the inscription of dependency on the old but syntactically reproducing the grammar of dependency in doing so. The case in point is a polemic by Richard Kalish (1981) against certain advocates for the elderly who, by representing the care needs of the least independent members of the group as typical of the whole, promote a stigmatic image of old age. Built into what Kalish calls the "new ageism" in gerontology are failure and incompetence accounts of the actual elderly, projected against a normative "geriactivist model" of the ideal elderly. Such accounts, Kalish protests, imply that the older person is "not only victimized, but is also impotent and powerless to have any significant impact on the society and/or individuals who perpetrate the victimization" (p. 237). To escape these undue extremes of criterial activism and proclamations of actual passivity and impotence—yet without abandoning a normative concept of good old age in the process—Kalish proposes a "personal growth model" whereby the later years "can be a period of optimum personal growth" (p. 239), with allowance being made for physical, financial, and other objective limitations, so as to be reasonable.

The point I want to make is that the conclusion of Kalish's polemic against rendering the elderly a passive, impotent, dependent population reproduces in its syntax an us–them power division between ourselves and the elderly, together with an underlying conferment on them of passivity and impotence:

> *We* can develop a Personal Growth model, so that *we can approach* older persons with the expectation that *they* have the potential for continued growth, that even sickness and financial restriction can be a source of growth, although not desirable, and that *our* task is to facilitate that growth. *We can communicate to* older persons that we have faith in their abilities, that *we recognize* that *they* are capable of making decisions (even those decisions that *we assume*, perhaps correctly, will turn out wrong), that *we respect* their ownership of their own bodies and times and lives. In brief *we can communicate* a Success Model instead of the Failure Models. (Kalish, 1981:241 emphases added)

The voice is benevolent and humane but the utterances, by their shape, could only be about a dependent population (the term "older persons" could, for example, be replaced by "children," "prisoners," "mental patients," or "native peoples" without loss of intelligibility), and they are delivered from a standpoint of power–knowledge beyond those referred to. The "older persons" are not part of the "we" that recognizes and communicates how best to be old. They are made objects of an address from outside and above, subjected in discourse to criterial concepts prescribed and delivered by others, just as in social policy the aged are targeted recipients of care services "prescribed and provided" by others (Estes, 1979:5). Reproduction of the grammar of dependence, if only in syntax, produces effects of power–knowledge dependency, regardless of intent. When, therefore, Estes (1979) attacks "age-segregated policies . . . that single out, stigmatize, and isolate the aged from the rest of society" (p. 5), she needs also to be heard as attacking age-segregating discursive practices that do the same thing. When she subtitles her study a "Critical Examination of Social Policies and Services for the Aged," this should be heard, for the sake of critical completeness, as including the syntax of dependency echoed in the subtitle itself. Language effects are too important, and too insidious, to be taken for granted.

THE PLACE OF KINDNESS IN THE GRAMMAR
OF CARE AND DEPENDENCY

It is said that care waits to be answered by dependency, but kindness needs no answer. If this is so we must ask what place, if any, kindness has in the care–dependency circuit of gerontological discourse. Can it have any exchange value in this economy of terms when it seems so obviously to be excluded? I will argue that it does, but only if kindness is understood in a certain way. A way exorbitant to ordinary usage.

In ordinary use, kindness signifies a moral sentiment, feeling or disposition toward others. It would be absurd, i.e., ungrammatical, to speak of a *system* of kindness, *organized provision* of kindness, a *continuum* of kindness, or kindness professionals, whereas it is perfectly grammatical to speak in these ways of care. Due, I would suggest, to grammatical limitations on incorporating 'kindness' into scientifically and instrumentally rational discourse, the term has no regular place in the lexicon of gerontology and hardly ever surfaces in the literature. It cannot, however, be simply ignored since it is culturally close to caring for or about others, and gerontology is bound also to display cultural as well as scientific and instrumental intelligibility. This is where the exorbitant meaning of the term enters.

Ordinary language dictionaries place kindness under the term *kind*, which, as a noun, means of the same sort; hence derivatives such as kin and kindred. The adjective *kind* is defined by *Chambers Twentieth-Century Dictionary* (1972) as "having or springing from the feelings natural for those of the same family." Tangentially, then, kindness can be understood as a type of contact relationship or contact structure. It may or may not contain the corresponding sentiment (there are, after all, unnatural feelings between kinsfolk as the literature on elder abuse testifies). To capture this structural, relational meaning I will refer to kind-ness. My argument is that in this sense, though under other names, kind-ness is incorporated into the continuum of care and so into the care—dependency circuit at the center of gerontology. My interest is in describing its discursive role and significance in the field.

Clear expressions of the idea of kind-ness appear in accounts of informal (versus formal or institutional) care. A good example is a paper by Litwak (1980) on the role of community mental health centers in helping the elderly. The centers embody a policy of help based on a fundamental distinction between "natural support systems," referring to primary groups, and "large-scale" institutions, characterized by formal organization (Litwak, 1980:80). Supplementary distinctions are made between services "tailored" to individual idiosyncracy and "standardized" services belonging to the "routinization of life" (p. 81), between "noninstrumental" and "instrumental" relationships to those being helped (p. 83), and between "nontechnical" and "technical" tasks of care (p. 84).

Two uses of kind-ness are evident in Litwak's discussion. One is to specify, conceptually and practically, the continuum of care via which gerontology, in its literary production practices, brings the elderly to rational comprehension. Standardized, instrumental care is so different from nonstandardized, noninstrumental care that "it is generally wise to separate the structures for handling technical tasks . . . from those handling idiosyncratic and nontechnical tasks . . . to separate the formal and the natural system" (Litwak, 1980:84). This does not mean, however, reducing the continuum of care to a dichotomy, which would be a reduction of scientific and instrumental rationality, but assigning tasks on the continuum of care to a continuum of institutions rather than trying to combine them in a single setting. In mental health care there has to be room for "half-way houses," group homes, and community mental health centers between "closed institutions" and "natural support systems" (p. 118). Between, that is, lifeworld kind-ness of family, friends, and community, and categorial, classificatory kind-ness designed for treatment, supervision, and administration. From this it is obvious that the role of kind-ness in specifying way-stations along the continuum of care, thus contributing to the technical representation of elderliness in gerontology, is by no means confined to the particular instance of mental health.

A second use of kind-ness, already intimated above, is to conduct rhetorics of regret, shame, rebuke, repair, and renewal. Litwak, while admitting the necessity of institutional care, speaks with feeling of the virtues of noninstrumental, nontechnical, noneconomic contact structures, of the "deep, personal involvement" (p. 83) and respect for idiosyncracy they allow for. Along the same lines of commonplace contrast (the kind of contrast essential for displaying cultural rationality in social science), Treas (1981:327) rebukes those who accuse people of abandoning their older kinsfolk and leaving care to the state and formal institutions: "a discordant lament is heard for the passing of filial piety in America. An oft-voiced sentiment holds that young people no longer accord the parental generation the respect, love, and help that are traditionally its due. Indeed, some would blame the indifference of kin for the social isolation and economic insecurity confronting so many of the aged." The accusation, which is one of lost or disappearing natural kindness and its substitution by formal replacements, is said to be unfair.

Treas points out that due to demographic trends, there are fewer kin to provide elders, now longer-living, with support: "fewer descendents to call upon for assistance" (p. 329), "a shortage of 'maiden aunts' to devote themselves to parents" (p. 331). Apart from objective shrinkage in kinship networks there is no evidence that they are any less caring. As to the substitution of formal for family care (categorial for natural kind-ness), gerontologists are finding complementarity rather than replacement. Social programs are said to have "created a new role for kin as mediators between institutional bureaucracies and elderly relations" (p. 327). Finally, such replacement as does occur is instrumentally rational and intersubjectively reasonable: "No longer are the children of these 'frail elderly' prime-age adults. The very old in greatest need of care have offspring who are the 'young–old' with their declining energy, health, and finances" (p. 330). Also, even the most devoted kin cannot supply specialized treatment, "daily ministrations," and "custodial care" (p. 335). These are matters for "a service industry and a professional corps" (p. 335).

The truth, adequacy, or validity of these statements is not the issue here. All I am concerned to establish is the role of the concept of kindness (encoded in terms like "family," "children", "offspring," and "filial piety") in motivating and composing such statements—in making them possible. Its role, to put it more broadly, in joining scientific and instrumental formulations of the nature and significance of aging to ordinary language formulations, thus allowing the grammar of care to be performed in all three registers of rationality.

Treas's references to past compared to present conditions point to a third usage of kind-ness in gerontology: the fashioning of narratives about care from the possibilities provided by its grammar. Narrative is another constitutive feature of cultural rationality and the accountable orderliness of human affairs, consequently it is a requisite feature of intelligible reconstructions of social reality. (For detailed arguments along these lines, see, Habermas, 1979b; White, 1980; Ricoeur, 1981; Danto, 1985; Polkinghorne, 1988.)

A fine example of narrative usage is Quadagno's (1986) excavation of historical legacies informing present American programs for old age security. Her reconstruction of early colonial provisions for old age dependency describes care structures based on family and community kind-ness. The aged were cared for under the same rules of responsibility as the poor, those of "local responsibility, family responsibility, and the residency requirement of legal settlement" (p. 130). The last rule was to ensure that only bona fide members of the community were included under its care, excluding those of another kind. One practice of local responsibility was for old people to assign their property to the community in return for lifetime care, showing how residentially authenticated kind-ness could be turned into old age security in a relatively closed society of people known to each other.

Changes in public provisions of care include a narrative of "increased impersonality of public relief" (Quadagno, 1986:133) as county and state bureaucracies took over from local communities, with countervailing efforts to preserve care structures of kind-ness, or invent new ones. For example, Quadagno relates that one response was for "some groups, on the basis of national origin or religious ties, to form charitable organizations, soliciting funds in anticipation of need" (p. 133). There were mutual aid societies based on ethnic and religious rather than family and residential kind-ness, but continuous with them. Achenbaum (1978:42) observes: "After the Civil War, more and more denominations and ethnic groups had established private old-age homes. The aim was to provide a home-like setting for the elderly, particularly those without kith or kin."

Further to the significance of "kind-ness" in gerontology and the semiolinguistic value of its terms, Laslett (1985) warns against the empirical dubiousness of strong contrasts between a past (before industrialization and capitalism), when the aged had a positive place in a society organized around primary groups, and a present position of inactive marginality in large-scale, impersonal structures. Such contrasts lead to the construction of Edenic mythologies, where "the deficiencies of the present are referred to the destruction of an idealized society" (p. 204), rather than accurate histories of aging. What needs to be added, however, is that the concept of kind-ness has a role in gerontology beyond making statements about past and present realities, and beyond, therefore, purely empirical valuation. This role is to construct, rehearse, and debate policy options, leading gerontology into questions of how aging is done rather than what it is.

Quadagno points toward the encoding of divergent rationales of care in her concluding remarks about the history of old age security. Referring to the principle of local responsibility and the exclusion of strangers from it, she remarks that although the principle allowed for "personalized care" it also made care difficult to administer: "The principle of local responsibility was simply inapplicable to a growing nation, a nation increasingly composed of strangers who could not simply be 'warned away'" (Quadagno, 1986:149). Care by kind-ness is not, however, an option (a rationale) that has been closed off by the passage of time. It survives, as we have seen, in efforts to make room in administered care for "natural support systems." It survives also in a policy question posed by Quadagno: "Should social security function primarily as an insurance program, returning benefits to individuals on the basis of past contributions? Or should income be redistributed to equalize social inequities by paying benefits on the basis of need?" (p. 150).

Underlying these options is a contrast between two ways of rationalizing administered care. One, corresponding to Quadagno's second question, is near to care by kind-ness; the other is distant and removed from it. One is based on particularistic relationships to others (kinship, friendship, community), and the other on universalistic relationships (juridical contract, associational membership, financial contract). One conveys rightful care to fellow members on the basis of likeness, and the other conveys rightful care to individual citizens, clients, purchasers on the basis of a legally valid claim of entitlement (for example, payment for services, a record of insurance or pension plan contributions, a citizenship certificate).

In societies stressing the value of individual responsibility, such as the United States, those whose entitlement claims leave them short of care must have recourse to formally defined collective kind-ness (public welfare), a denigrated alternative, to make up the deficit. Such recourse is marked by degradation ceremonies (for example, the suspicion procedures of welfare offices) to display deviance from moral desirability, thus turning financial problems into a social plight.

In societies stressing collective responsibility, where the public sphere is social democratic rather than liberal democratic in organization, care is an aspect of national membership, a right of kind-ness at the national level. The contemporary emblem of a social democratic society, and a frequently occupied place of discourse in gerontology, is Sweden. Paul Friday (1981) makes typical use of the place in describing a society that regards itself as the home of a unitary folk community and "citizens as members of one family in that home" (p. 131). Szemberg (1988:12) says that "the political culture of Sweden is defined by two notions: *folkhem* (people's home) and *trygghet* (shelter, security)." Consistent with the particularistic logic of care by kind-ness, which keeps out strangers, Sweden has until recently remained remarkably free of "foreign" elements.

The question of whether these are empirically accurate statements about a real place called Sweden is not at issue here. What is important is that the meaning space of that name represents a way of doing care—particularistic care based on commitments of kind-ness—that can be contrasted with another way—universalistic care based on contractual obligation—and thus provide for argumentation about programs and policy options. Characterizations of the past as a place of kind-ness different from the present serve the same discursive function. I would emphasize, however, that the contrasts, no matter how strongly or critically made, remain within the care–dependency circuit of discourse and its grammar of usage. Proposals for change, reform, restructuring, rethinking, redefinition, and the like have to be made within those bounds because they are conditions for rendering old age a reader-recognizeable reality in rational discourse, which is to say, rational for us in our form of social life. Change beyond those bounds would have to be a change of the bounds—a change in the structure of rational recognition—a task that is, by definition, beyond the scope of rational discourse and deliberate planning, since these *are* the bounds.

CHAPTER

4

Mechanisms of Field Organization in Gerontology

In Chapter 2, I described the emergence of a virtual field of study of old age from diverse practices of knowledge production. The present chapter analyses the discursive means through which gerontology occupies the field and turns a possible into an actual area of study. Occupancy is the central theme of the chapter. It is to be understood, however, as a continuous operation performed on each and every occasion that gerontology is done, not as a once and finished historical act of invasion and seizure. Gerontology is done, like every intellectual discipline, in local acts of language use; it continuously accomplishes and reproduces its distinctive order of thought in linguistic acts of settlement and extension across a region of possible meanings.

To bring these geopolitical metaphors to bear on discourse analysis, I will rely on three concepts drawn from literary and language studies: *appropriation*, *specification*, and *articulation*. I take appropriation to be the basic activity and the others auxiliaries of it.

There is one more preparatory point to be made before defining and applying the concepts. The emphasis of this chapter is on the integration and orderliness of the field. This is not to say, however, that disintegrative tendencies and internal contradictions are lacking or less important. Indeed they belong to the order of the field itself. What Simmel said of performatively real rather than merely formal integration in social groups holds also for a field of discourse: "society, in order to attain a determinate shape, needs some quantitative ratio of harmony and disharmony, of association and competition, of favorable and unfavorable tendencies. But these discords are by no means mere sociological liabilities or negative instances. Definite, actual society does not result only from other social forces which are positive, and only to the extent that the negative factors do not hinder them" (Simmel, 1971:72). Sources of discord in gerontology include, as we have seen, conflict between the performative requirements of scientific and cultural rationality. More deeply, they also include conflict between the aim of discourse to achieve security of meaning and the immanent insecurity generated by

105

the semiotic movement of language from sign to sign: the dialectic of discourse and text. These features of field organization are to be examined in the following chapter.

APPROPRIATION OF THE SUBJECT-MATTER

I will begin by amplifying some points made in the methodology chapter concerning the role of basic categories designating the subject matter of a discipline. The role, that is, of legisigns in establishing an order of discourse.

Fields of social inquiry are composed of a tremendous variety of linguistic materials: semantic elements from the linguistic life of society, ideological formulas, institutional accounting practices, and relevant knowledges from arts, sciences, and technologies. We have already seen this to be the case with gerontology. Such diversity opens up a prospectively overwhelming proliferation of discursive possibilities. Discipline occupancy of a field is based on a methodical delimitation of possibilities: an ordering of sentence-propositions into repeated sets, circuits, and patterns and a placement of inscriptive design on the semiolinguistic materials of the field. Crucial in achieving this is the conceptual condensation of the field into a subject matter named by a master category, or by a close cluster of categories, so that it can be said, "This [the name of the discipline] is the study of . . . [the master category or cluster]." Disciplinary propositions (definitions, descriptions, axioms, hypotheses, and so on) are then required to stem from and return to the master category or cluster, either directly or through explicable detours. To say that a particular discipline is *about* a particular master category, as, for example, gerontology is about aging and the aged, is not merely a formal definition of its content but a description of its discursive composition and linguistic architecture.

To fill out the concept of appropriation it is helpful to recall, through Weimann (1988), that although the English term has become fairly narrowly associated with private property and juridical possession (connotations that I certainly wish to preserve in the idea of a field legisign), its German counterpart, *Aneignung*, has broader and more active meanings. These are exploited by Karl Marx in referring to the appropriation of natural materials through working on them. It can be further pointed out that Marx was appropriating the political economists' master categories of "use value" and "exchange value" for his own critical purpose. As Weimann says, appropriation can be linked to intellectual and literary acts of representation: "In regard to the functions of representation, then, appropriation would have to be defined at the intersection of both text-appropriating and world-appropriating activities. . . . These activities will be conceived in terms of *Aneignung*, of making things (relations, books, texts, writings) one's own" (Weimann, 1988:433). In my terms, the distinction between text-appropriating and world-appropriating activities refers, within a field of discourse, to the production, respectively, of knowledge effects and reality effects, the latter being representations of the world outside the field pointed to by its legisigns. Knowledge effects are produced in disciplinary appropriations of real world representations. A field of discourse is, therefore, a redoubling appropriation of internal text and contextual world in one. Legisigns are gathering places in the surface of a field where these two moments of appropriative activity intersect.

The legisigns, and master categories, of gerontology are *aging* and *the aged*. Of these, "the aged" is especially important because of its stronger "world-appropriating" capacity. This can be related to its grammatical status as a substantive noun and, in comparison, the status of aging as a present participle combining the functions of verb and adjective. (Aging is a consort legisign related more to articulating the subject matter of the field than to its direct appropriation.)

Posner (1982), seeking rules to explain why certain sequences of adjectives before nouns are preferred to alternatives—seeming more natural, grammatical, and meaningful—invokes the criterion of variability. Adjectives less open to interpretation, less in need of comparisons to specify their meaning, and with a smaller number of relata will be closer to a noun, both in sequential order and in security of meaning, than more open adjectives. For example, *frail, old lady* is grammatically and intuitively preferable to *old, frail lady* because the interpretation of *old* rests on fewer processing moves than that of *frail*; it has a more nominal character. The preferred sequence conforms to the rule that "local proximity to the head noun indicates nouniness" (Posner, 1982:60). To explicate the connection of low–high variability of meaning to the noun–adjective distinction, Posner introduces Aristotle's distinction between "substances" and "accidentals": "nouns designate substances and attribute adjectives designate accidentals" (1982:71). Posner's elaboration of the comparison makes it clear why "the aged" is appropriatively stronger in discourse than "aging." A noun determines its designation in and of itself, rather than through being comparatively related to other terms, and the designata of head nouns remain relatively constant, functioning to preserve referential identity in the midst of adjectival variability and replacement.

These observations on the stronger "world-appropriating" capacity of "the aged" than "aging" can be reinforced by considering the other grammatical element of the term: the definite article *the*. Hamilton

(1949:8) observes that "the definite article in its normal use points to an object, imagined or conceived, which can be *recognized*, whether or no it has been mentioned before" (emphasis added). The definite article induces an effect of immediate recognition, being in this respect functionally equivalent to a prior plausibility structure. To speak of "the aged," therefore, implies common knowledge of something already known between writer and reader, as well a substantively existent object beyond both. The reading effect of *the* plus a noun is to claim objective credibility for whatever is named within the bounds of a world already known in common. It is a linguistic structure eminently suited to meet the requirements of both scientific and cultural rationality, of discipline and societal membership. It is a cognitive and recognitional device all in one.

The cognitive function of a legisign is to bring conceptual order to details, particulars, and otherwise isolated representations of reality. It is illustrated in Garfinkel's case study of Suicide Prevention Center workers attached to the Coroner's Office in Los Angeles (Garfinkel, 1967:11–18). Their job is to conduct a "psychological autopsy" on cases of sudden death that are equivocal between suicide and some other cause (homicide, accident, or natural cause). In effect, they search through the evidence of a case, the remnants of a life, the whatsoever bits and pieces, to see if they can be brought under the governance of the legisign *suicide* and thereby rendered accountable deaths; if not, then whether they can be seen as replicas in detail of one of the other death categories. Garfinkel's description is especially useful in making it clear that the categories do not function as passive boxes into which things are sorted but as active scanning devices that *make* things known and *organize* particulars into conceptual structures. Ricoeur (1977:105) similarly argues that the primary function of a concept is "to recognize the individual nature of the object, not to constitute general attributes," adding that the function is especially suited to "the use of the substantive in language, prior to qualities or actions being brought to it by means of adjectives and verbs." Subsequently Ricoeur cites a neglected scholar, Hedwig Konrad, on the role of a substantive noun in determining for thought the structural arrangement of an object's representations and in defining its essential structure of attributes. Konrad calls this selective articulation of attributes defining the object "the fundamental order of the concept" (Ricoeur, 1977:339). When the noun in question is a field legisign, then the fundamental order of the concept is simultaneously a fundamental order of the whole field of discourse whose subject matter the noun grasps.

Fowler (1981) adds a consideration crucial to our theme. He points to the nominalization of verbs characteristic of legal, administrative, and technical documents as cases of broader linguistic processes: the "lexicalization" and "relexicalization" of ordinary language. Lexicalization refers to special language formations, arcane to the uninitiated, in trades, professions, and among hobbyists, technicians, street gangs, etc. Relexicalization compounds the process. Fowler's point is that nouns are especially suited to these in-folding complications of social discourse. The social sciences, to their own uneasiness, have become advance guards of relexicalization.

The preceding arguments relate especially in gerontology to "the aged," but to the extent that its consort, "aging," is nominalized through repeated conjunctions with head nouns (as in "the aging process" and "aging populations"), it acquires a comparable appropriative capacity.

The scale and reach of these categories in articulating a gerontological order of discourse among manifold details are impressive. Their range of inscription extends from body tissues to census tables, and from institutional ceremonies of passage to familiar minutiae of everyday life. Biologists have inscribed AGE (advanced glycosylation end product) acronymically in molecular protein changes related to "the stiffening and loss of elasticity characteristic of aging tissues" (Cerami et al., 1987:90). Medical researchers inscribe aging symptomatically in reaction time decreases, reduced cardiovascular efficiency, reduced renal blood flow, hearing problems, sight disorders, rheumatism, and digestive problems. Psychologists inscribe aging in measures of memory performance, information processing, and mental health; sociologists inscribe it in role loss, patterns of interaction, and provisions of care services. Care workers find signs of old age in mundane behaviors such as dawdling: "the tendency of older residents in institutions to return from an activity so slowly that they require supervision" (Harris, 1988:48), and in speaking about the past: "a commonly noted activity among the elderly is reminiscing, which many people associate with senility and living in the past" (Cormican, 1980:252). The power of categories to make connections between manifold things, to synthesize details into a subject matter, thereby appropriating them and making them available for discursive recognition, is amply demonstrated in the legisigns of gerontology. There is no researchable, discussable old age in the manifold of reality unless categories of language inscribe it there.

The appropriative operations of a field are not confined to the manifold of reality, they must also include prior means of representing the reality the field would make its own. In particular, where social science is concerned, there must be an appropriation of preexisting vocabularies, explanatory formulas, interpretive schemas, common place recipes, and so on from the ordinary and administrative languages of social life. Discipline field work necessarily includes sifting, sorting, absorbing, modifying, correcting, rejecting, and otherwise asserting normative authority over prior language use: a subordination of the language *of* social reality to a lexicalized language *about* it. This is necessary, first, to objectify social reality (which is done by fashioning an observation platform from its own semiolinguistic materials), and, second, to ensure the identity of a given text—in the course of being read—as a work of social science.

The point I would make here is that social science can only be done and, more importantly, can only be seen to be done in continuously working with and against prior languages of social life. The intent to do social science can be announced in titles, headings, and the like, but its actual performance occurs in moments and sequences of interpretive activity, an activity I am saying that moves between continuity with ordinary language and disciplinary appropriation of it. Calls to return social science to ordinary language miss the constitutive necessity of this movement, as do calls to abandon ordinary language completely. Even judicious calls to combine ordinary with mathematical language, creating parallel sets of meanings "saying the same thing in two ways" (Jasso, 1988:8) miss the constitutive necessity of working in and against ordinary language. Bilingual redundancy can no more satisfy this performative requirement of social science than unilingual reduction.

The necessity of interweaving technical and ordinary language can be argued also through the concept of membership. A social science text, to be performatively such in an act of reading, needs to hold the reader in a dual membership: membership of a society known in common, unremarkably providing referential sense to text statements, and membership of a specialized knowledge community cognitively coordinate and superordinate to ordinary membership. The requirement is met through inserting discipline-specific language practices into those of ordinary language and in strategically crucial moments of methodological authority replacing them. (For example, replacing common place words with formal definitions, operational definitions, and testable hypothoses.) In these ways, which are ways of scripting reading performances, referential contents of societal membership are appropriated as the topical subject matter of a discipline. Since it is only in such work (i.e., text work) of appropriation that social science can be seen to be done, it cannot be dispensed with. Therefore every field must have the characteristic structure of a discipline lexicon directing a multiple organization of ordinary and other operative language elements of social life.

In gerontology, as in other "recent," "new," and "immature" fields of social science, the establishment of linguistic authority is a salient problem. Conversely, signs of its salience provide the evident sense of terms such as immaturity of the field. One such sign evident in the topical organization of gerontology is a concern to identify myths, misconceptions, and common errors in prior formulations of its subject matter. In terms of an earlier discussion (Chapter 2), this is an attempt to draw borderlines, that is, simultaneous connections and divisions, with the foundational sources of the field. Some illustrations will help further describe the organizational dynamics of gerontology as an order of discourse.

Novak (1988) is representative of the field in defining the goal of academic gerontology as the erasure of "prejudice and stereotyping in society by writing about the facts of aging," and in comparing "myths and the facts that gerontologists have found to replace them" (Novak, 1988:9). The myths all have to do with beliefs of loss, deficit, and victimization—loss of social contacts, deficits of functional capacity, liability to criminal victimization—as do those collected by Palmore (1977) and incorporated into a true–false quiz, every statement of which rings common sensically true but is, in gerontological fact, false. The pedagogy is the same as Durkheim's opening to the study of suicide—a work that is itself a demarcation of the new science of sociology—namely, a demonstration from the standpoint of a disciplinary "we" that what we in general know to be true is in fact false. The contrast structure of ironic reversal is typical of a new discipline wanting to make its way and establish its place in the social world, something that can be done only by representing mundane representations from a higher cognitive stance. It is, moreover, a structure of representation that social science writing is condemned to repeat because of the scientifically dubious gift of eternal youth, whereby its texts have to be rewritten, thus reborn, in new generational contexts. Shanas (1979) calls belief in the breakdown of family support for old people a "hydra-headed myth" that no amount of factual refutation can slay. Marshall (1987:262) remarks of the same belief: "Among those in the research community, myth destruction has reached the point of acute boredom, yet popular opinion, nourished by the popular media, persists in the view that the family is a social institution near collapse." A note of thankfulness rather than complaint would have been in order here. If gerontology was capable of once and for all replacing myths with facts it would eliminate the difference between societal and disciplinary membership knowledge, eliminate boundary transactions across that difference, and thus eliminate its own indispensable source of nourishment. It would dry into an uninhabitable desert of pure discourse without boundary, limit, or point.

The status of social science as knowledge about "knowledge," i.e., metaknowledge, is evident in the myth–fact contrast. It is reinforced when previous contrasts come to be included as data in higher order judgments. For example, the National Council on Aging, an advocacy group for older Americans, sponsors what are called Myth and Reality of Aging surveys, but gerontologists submit the results to their own methodological criteria to ensure that they are not myths in extra disguise. Montgomery et al. (1987:168) include the surveys as a data set to be critically appropriated, placing them at the threshhold of gerontology along with other societal sources of knowledge. The same trajectory of higher order inclusion is enacted by Laslett (1985) when he adduces "painfully recovered facts" (p. 209) to reveal that accepted knowledge claims about dramatic changes in the situation of the aged after the advent of modern, industrial society are, in fact, "dogmas" lodged in "informal theorization" and reflections of "quasi-theoretical assumptions" corresponding to "popular attitudes" (p. 201). All the quoted terms are, like "myth," representations of false, lacking, or only partial knowledge: mere appearances of the real thing.

From the standpoint of the literary production of knowledge effects, it is relevant that Laslett's terms form an immediately recognizable order of progressive inclusion and replacement: from popular attitudes, through quasitheoretical assumptions and informal theorizing, to painfully recovered facts, and, in anticipation, "formal theory" (Laslett, 1985:201). There is something about the order itself that is immediately credible and that, in the reading experience, confers a presumption of incremental credibility on the unfolding text quite in advance of logical or factual persuasion. It has something like the effect of a chronologically ordered review of the literature at the beginning of a research monograph. It seems in its very shape and structure to be emblematic of knowledge.

A possible explanation lies in the concept of "iconicity in syntax" suggested by Posner (1982). In Charles Peirce's semiotics an icon is a type of sign that communicates a designatum by means of structural analogy. Maps and diagrams are examples. Posner argues that the sequential, spatial, syntactic organization of sentences is normally taken to be a narrative or logical order belonging to their referential meaning. Properties of sentence organization are transferred to the designatum. We previously considered the case where the relative proximity of two or more adjectives to a head noun conveys both their relative semantic closeness to the particular noun and their relative linguistic closeness to the properties of nouns in general. Posner's level of analysis is unduly abstract and technical for our purpose but his reference to the coding of narrative order in syntactic structure plus his observation (p. 51) that "iconic text interpretation" is a function not only of natural language competence but a particular reading attitude and, presumably, membership of a definite reading community, allows movement to another level: that of cultural and discourse analysis. Here I would argue that for the

reader in a field of social science there exists a narrative that in its very
form certifies credibility and gives the imprimatur of knowledge. It is a
narrative about science, the metonymic touchstone of knowledge in our
culture, which Rorty (1980) calls the "up the mountain" story.

The story tells of error left behind and below in a laborious but steady
climb toward truth. Its certifying power is obviously related to the rational and charismatic authority of its natural science provenance. Rorty's
title, however, calls attention to another source: the connection of the
story to some of the metaphors we think by in ordinary language. Lakoff
and Johnson (1980:Ch. 4) identify a series of "orientational metaphors,"
based on physical and cultural experiences of space, which organize
entire systems of concepts, that is fundamental orders of discourse in
everyday knowledge. Among these are metaphors of verticality directly
relevant to the "up the mountain" story: good is up, bad is down; conscious is up, unconscious is down (one wakes *up* and *falls* asleep); rational is up, emotional is down (discussion is *raised* to a higher level by
leaving emotion *behind*). Further to the metaphor "rational is up," Lakoff
and Johnson observe that references to low-level (or, we might add,
immature) science are based on the metaphor "mundane reality is
down" (Lakoff and Johnson, 1980:19). Performative distancing from the
ordinary language formulations of mundane reality is, therefore, a positive upward movement toward rational consciousness even within the
frame of ordinary orientational metaphors. It is even more strongly so
within the frame of the "up the mountain" story of knowledge.

A stretch of discourse that begins with statements of myth, popular
opinion, common belief, or dogma and successively supplements them
with discipline statements of fact and logic is not only telling the story of
knowledge in its content but is reproducing the structure of the story in
its syntactic organization. Iconic replication thus combines with story
content to form a strong appropriation device. It is a device that in
literarily taking over terms from ordinary and other operative languages
of social life produces reading effects of cumulative knowledge. At the
moment of reading, the next statement in such a device is presumptively
higher up the mountain than the last, hence, in prospect, more credible
and knowledgeable. The "up the mountain" story enters reading as an
interpretive posture, the disciplinary functions of which are to appropriate a subject matter and confer authority on a field.

In conclusion, gerontology must, as a condition of disciplinary existence, include, encompass, and textually appropriate ordinary language
formulations of aging and the aged. When Durkheim (1983:91) says that
"scientific thought cannot rule alone" and that there will always be room
for "a form of truth which will perhaps be expressed in a very secular
way, but will nevertheless have a mythological . . . basis," he could well

be stating a rule of social scientific writing: a rule of the genre. This seems not to be the case because almost immediately, in the same passage, Durkheim calls the joint operation of scientific truth and mythological truth in social life "one of the great obstacles which obstruct the development of sociology" (1983:91). Yet this was not his final word on the subject. In his last book, *The Elementary Forms of the Religious Life*, Durkheim explores the social origins of thought and offers this comment on science:

> So opinion, primarily a social thing, is a source of authority, and it might even be asked whether all authority is the daughter of opinion. It may be objected that science is often the antagonist of opinion, whose errors it combats and rectifies. But it cannot succeed in this task if it does not have sufficient authority, and it can obtain this authority only from opinion itself. (Durkheim, 1915:238–239)

The "hydra-headed" myth referred to by Shanas (1979) is not simply an emblem of error, it represents everyday language in all its fertile proliferation, and it should be spoken of with gratitude—as Durkheim came to do—not as a monster to be slain, since it is in and against this proliferation that social science takes shape.

The dialectic of scientific and everyday language is further displayed in the other two mechanisms of field organization to be considered: specification and articulation.

SPECIFICATION OF THE SUBJECT-MATTER

The work of specification is to grasp and pin down the subject matter of a field in stable grids of utterance. It is thus continuous (as pointed out in Chapter 1) with one meaning of articulation: to give utterance. Specification, however, plays a distinctive role in the organization of a field that warrants separate consideration. The role is to give objective reference to the legisigns of a field, the master categories through which an entire subject matter is collected and relayed. In gerontology, these categories being aging and the aged.

To appreciate the work we need to recall that in everyday usage the terms aging and the aged have open, shifting applications whose definiteness depends on who is using them, how, when and where. In other words, their meaning is indexical to circumstantial actions. To make them the governing categories of a field demands, then, special care. Used ordinarily they might import into gerontology the "intellectual chaos" discerned by Homans (1961:1) in everyday generalizations about

social behavior, a chaos arising from their merely ad hoc grasp of reality
and the fact that "nobody tries to put them together" (p. 2). Sacks
(1989:366) remarks that Homans' complaint, a standard way of opening
a social science text, is not against chaos but against ad hoc rationality
and what might be called the "atopical" organization of knowledge (p.
372). This is knowledge lodged in maxims, proverbs, and the like,
whose validity is immediately recognized in local acts and contexts of
application. It is different, therefore, from knowledge lodged in propositional statements, the validity of which depends on empirical and logical
assessment. Assessment, that is, through methodically traversing topics
stated and implied in statements about reality. The work of specification
can be described then as one of abstracting atopical formations of knowledge from ordinary language and turning them into topical formations
of a discipline.

Another way to describe the work of specification is through Ricoeur's
account of the difference between the subjective and objective meaning
of discourse (Ricoeur, 1976:19–20). Objective meaning alludes to propositional content and the meaning encoded in sentence structure, while
the subjective side is what the utterer does and intends. Specification
works to standardize subjective meaning in a collective discipline lexicon and make referential meaning the entire meaning of utterances:
"The reference expresses the full exteriorization of discourse to the extent that the meaning is not only the ideal object intended by the utterer,
but the actual reality aimed at by the utterance" (Ricoeur, 1976:80).

Specification, in summary, fastens a subject matter to standard terminological grids, thus ensuring its repeated, shared availability to a
knowledge community; and it fastens interpretation to the exterior side
of language and referential interpretants of signs, thus making of language a plain channel of objective meaning. To further specify specification, it is helpful to introduce the distinction between conceptual and
operational grids made in Chapter 1. Whereas the former break down
master categories through theoretical models, classifications, and formal
schemas, the latter take the measure of a designated subject matter
through research instruments and through pragmatic paradigms of the
subject matter.

Pragmatic paradigms of aging and the aged have been discussed previously in relation to provisions for care and the societal foundations of
gerontology. They include residential classifications, the design of old
people's homes, and retirement rules. The numerous public programs
for older people—in America, for example, the Retired Senior Volunteer
Program, the Foster Grandparent Program, the Senior Companion Program, the Friendly Visitor Program, the Nutrition Program, the area
agency transportation programs, the Personal Care Assessment pro-

gram, the Handyman and Homemakers Services for the Elderly—are pragmatic grids of specification. The tremendous array of public provisions for the elderly referred to by Estes (1979) as "the aging enterprise," and by Gelfand and Olsen (1983) as "the aging network," is not just a service delivery system nor, as Estes argues, a stigmatic labeling apparatus (though it may reasonably be regarded as both), the provisions are also means for knowing the old and making old age a recognizable reality in social practice. The cognitive function of public programs, which is by no means confined to labeling or stereotyping, must also be considered.

Pragmatic paradigms are used in institutional settings as devices enabling members of those settings to describe, explain, justify, or otherwise make referential sense of their actions, and also to certify the pertinence of their actions—showing, say, that painting a wall or cooking a meal is caring for the elderly. They operate, that is, in the way ascribed by Wieder (1974) to "the convict code" in a halfway house, whereby the code generated an accountable social reality for staff, inmates, and the researcher alike. The way is that of the documentary method of interpretation (Garfinkel, 1967:76–103), whereby evident details and conceptual patterns are made mutually recognizeable in each other: the former as documentary instances of the conceptual pattern, and the latter as a virtual meaning realized in the details.

From the standpoint of a discipline and the immanent task of showing that what is being written is—in the case we are considering—gerontology, pragmatic paradigms are at the extrascientific margin of the field. To make the boundary visible, they cannot be simply repeated but must be discursively worked on and appropriated. The task at hand is, after all, doing gerontology, not doing social work, health care, or something else. Especially important here is the conceptual interpretation of pragmatic paradigms so that they are made documentary details of higher order patterns. The schematic model of services to older people developed by Cantor and Little (1985), and discussed previously in another context, provides an example.

In their diagram of the model, the elderly are surrounded by concentric circles representing support structures. The diagrammatic space signifies a conceptual progression from informal (inner) to formal (outer) structures: the progression being informal (primary), informal (secondary), quasiformal (tertiary), and formal structures. Government programs are located in an outer circle of formal structures, making them, and the pragmatic paradigms of old age they contain, into documentary indicators of the formal–informal pattern. As always, it is through an embedded lodging of mundane social knowledge within a hierarchical conceptual order that social science is done, and seen to be done.

The same documentary trajectory is illustrated by Lawton's (1985) account of residential decisions and the housing of older people. At the mundane level are people making familiar decisions if, when, and where to move. At a somewhat higher abstractive level—that of public institutional arrangements, public policy vocabularies, and pragmatic paradigms of old age—are types of housing: retirement villages, mobile home parks, congregate housing, echo housing, the accessory apartment, share-a-home, and so on. These two linguistic layers of social knowledge are then made into documentary instances of higher order (more abstract, stable, and exact) conceptual patterns through terms taken from and secured by disciplinary lexicons. Residential decisions reflect the older person's taking either "a proactive or a passive stance in relation to the environment" (Lawton, 1985:450). Housing types reflect an "independent-supportive environment continuum" (p. 461). Residential moves to and from housing types can be classified for comparative research purposes into amenity moves, environmental push moves, and assistance moves. It could be said that this is a relatively informal, ad hoc level of theorizing, but saying so only projects the same documentary method of knowledge production further ahead and thus reinforces the argument. In social science, it is the indexical connection of textually reproduced mundane detail with discursively composed conceptual pattern that founds knowledge, not the correspondence of things with words or data with hypotheses.

Pragmatic paradigms are closely tied to institutional practices at the margin of a field. As such they belong to the materials from which a discipline draws (and withdraws) cognitive authority as well as to the means of discipline appropriation. More clearly internal to a field and more definitely belonging to its means of appropriation are research instruments and measurement devices. Their role in specifying a subject matter is to referentially pin down concepts through operational definitions. This is sufficiently familiar from methodology textbooks to require no special comment. From the standpoint of appraising the applied (ethical and political) importance of gerontology, however, it is relevant to note the range and reach of its instrumental grasp. Every imaginable (i.e., culturally recognizeable) sign of being and becoming old is used to take the measure of the phenomenon. Harris's *Dictionary of Gerontology* includes the following: Cavan Activity Inventory (covering family, friends, leisure, and economic activity), Cavan Adjustment Rating Scales (two, 10-step scales of social participation, one for primary, the other for secondary relationships), Death Anxiety Scale (DAS), Index of Activities of Daily Living (ADL) (a scale focusing on the unaided performance of six "personal care" activities—eating, toileting, dressing, bathing, getting in and out of bed, and continence), GULHEMP profile (measuring seven components of functional age concerning physical, mental, and social capacities), Instrumental Activities of Daily Living Scale (IADL) (covering such activities as shopping, telephoning, and cooking), and Life Satisfaction Index (LSIA) (a "self-reporting instrument" about mood, attitude, and morale). To these can be added devices such as the penile strain gauge, for measuring sexual capacity. Through such devices the master categories of gerontology are specified to minutia of everyday life and physical condition.

Conceptual grids of specification in gerontology include extensive typologies, models, and theories of old age, spanning the three research areas of the field: the biomedical, psychosocial, and socioeconomic areas. An inventory would not particularly help advance the argument and, since the appropriative significance of theoretical models lies in articulating rather than just specifying a subject matter, they are better left to the next section. By way of example, however, I would point to conceptual grids that pin down the meaning of aging.

Basic to the field, and all its formal definitions, is a typological distinction between individual aging and population aging. Individual aging is specified through biomedical models such as cellular theory, molecular theory, free radical theory, selective inhibition theory, aging clock theory, and single organ theory (Novak, 1988:80–85; Harris, 1988:17,163); through psychological models of information processing, memory loss, functional disorders of personality, and organic disorders of the brain; and through sociological models such as disengagement theory, activity theory, and continuity theory (Harris, 1988:3,42,56). Population aging is specified through demographic grids such as the population pyramid— a bar graph that allows the researcher in a single glance to see the aging profile of a country in time and over time—and demographic transition theory (Harris, 1988:51).

Individual and population aging are conceptually integrated in grids representing a linkage of biological, biographical, sociological, and historiographical time: the times marked by passage across events in physical development, individual experience, and collective life. The most important example in gerontology is the concept of a cohort. A cohort refers to a number of people "who have experienced the same significant life event within a specified time period" (Harris, 1988:38). The event may be birth, yielding the standard demographic idea of a birth cohort visible in chronological population statistics, or it may be a normatively timed biographical event such as marriage, parenthood, or retirement—one of the markers on the "social clock" (Neugarten et al., 1965)—yielding marriage, parenthood, and other sociological cohorts. Finally, the event may be historical, placing the stamp of a "period effect" (Harris, 1988:134) on an entire birth cohort, and yielding a concept synonymous with generation (Harris, 1988:77), in the sense of an age group linked by life style, value pattern, or collective trauma.

From this it is apparent that the term cohort brings into single discursive focus biological, biographical, sociological, and historical marks of temporal passage. It forms a place (topos) through which diverse materials on individual and population aging can be coordinated and given a secure locus: "Thus, we can also speak of the aging of cohorts, which seems to offer an intermediate formulation between the aging of individuals and the aging of populations" (Myers, 1985:175).

Not only can we (gerontologists) speak, through "cohort," of macro- and micro-, objective and subjective, collective and individual aging all in one, thus locating the subject matter within constituent coordinates of social science, but we can do so analytically, hence with greater certainty. It was for reasons of referential security that Durkheim (1938:34–46) required the social scientist to sift through lay representations of a phenomenon under study in search of its general characteristics, ones that would abstract the phenomenon from the flux of appearances and represent it "from an aspect that is independent of . . . individual manifestations" (p. 45). The specification of a subject matter requires, in other words, that concrete descriptions of content be replaced by analytical descriptions of pattern, form, and structure. This is what a conceptual grid achieves.

Bengston et al. (1985) sift concrete descriptions of aging into maturation, cohort, and period effects: "Cohort is a surrogate for the influence of past events (conceptualized in terms of socialization) on attitudes or behaviors (as structured by life chances). Period is a surrogate for the influence of contemporary events on attitudes" (Bengston et al., 1985:307–308). The same process of analytic substitution is evident also in Riley (1985). A diagram of her model (this itself being the substitute of a substitution) represents cohorts as diagonal lines on a graph, the vertical coordinate of which represents individual age, and the horizontal coordinate historical time: "a cohort refers to people who are aging [together] along both these dimensions" (Riley, 1985:374). The analytic description of a cohort includes the idea that each one has unique characteristics due to historical events and period effects; also that cohorts vary in size and sociological composition, and that at any particular point on the historical continuum cohort groups are cross-sectionally arranged in certain relations of cooperation and separation, integration and conflict. These relations, however, are historically contingent: "Aging is not an immutable process . . . the persons in the older age strata today are very different from older persons in the past or in the future" (Riley, 1985:371).

The analytic model of a cohort allows multiple substantive descriptions of aging—individual and collective, current and historical—to be drawn into the referential orbit of a single concept. The analytic description provides a conceptual grid that serves as a matrix of meaning, a matrix within which discipline knowledge objects can be fashioned from diverse semantic materials. A conceptual grid is, in effect, an enunciative workplace for making discipline statements.

ARTICULATION OF THE SUBJECT-MATTER

Specification of the subject matter of gerontology settles gathering places of discourse amid the flux of institutionally and common sensically generated meanings of aging and the aged. Occupancy of the field requires a further step, however. Linguistic pathways must be established between settlements of meaning and across the topical diversity separating them such as to (1) form a system of discourse, and (2) endow whatever materials are included with accountable sense (recalling that accountable sense is relative to membership of a societal and not just a professionally expert language community).

The analysis to follow argues that the linguistic pathways of gerontology are formed from three operations: metaphorical expansions of the two field legisigns, aging and the aged, metonymic elaborations of the legisigns and of their metaphorical expansions, and the conferral of narrative pattern (narrativity) on any and all materials authorized by the legisigns and their metaphorical–metonymic surrogates.

These three mechanisms work together in the articulation process. Hayden White (1978:128) refers to metaphor and metonymy as two "modalities of language use," where a modality is a certain way "we construe fields . . . of phenomena in order to 'work them up' into possible objects of narrative representation and discursive analysis." I take White to mean that a field of discourse cannot be textually occupied either through literal repetition of its governing categories (the legisigns of the field), or by massively multiplying factual instances of the categories, which would only be a work of wandering instanciation and not a decisive act of occupancy. There must be a methodical extension and controlled spread of governing categories, and an ordered multiplication of theorized topics.

METAPHORIC AND METONYMIC ARTICULATION

I will treat metaphorical expansion and metonymic extension together, in spite of their basic differences as linguistic mechanisms, because they are so closely interwoven in discursive practice. There is a kind of lockstitch arrangement whereby the metaphorical reframing of a topic, for example, old age, shifts discourse sideways to another chain of metonymic associations. Since metaphor is the primary means of topic expansion, I will make this the focus of analysis. The particular metaphors to be examined—the dominant metaphors of the field—are the aged is a social class, the aged is a minority group, aging is deficit accumulation, aging is a journey, aging is a passage, aging is a life cycle, and aging is a support convoy. Because of their closeness the last four metaphors will be considered together.

Prior to the analysis, some observations are in order concerning the meaning of metaphor and metonymy. They are so surrounded with debate (see, for example, Ortony, 1979), particularly metaphor, that a position needs to be stated on the issues that have emerged.

To begin, I take a relatively narrow, technical view of metaphor rather than equating it loosely with all figurative language or, even more loosely, with language per se. Metaphor has a distinctive linguistic structure carrying distinctive language effects, the most important of which for discourse are effects of reality and knowledge.

Metaphor renames something and, in doing so, predicates something about it. The linguistic structure of metaphor corresponds to the particular way it does renaming, which is through analogical equivalence. Metonymy also renames, without, however, making a predicative statement because it only replaces one word with another. Also, it renames on the basis of experiential association, instrumental linkage, and spatiotemporal proximity rather than analogical equivalence. A metaphor, being analogically constructed, states an equivalence between two units. These are variously referred to by language theorists as the primary object and the secondary subject (Black, 1979), topic and vehicle, topic and comment, or tenor and vehicle (Ortony, 1979:1–16). The primary subject, or topic, is carried into the secondary subject by an assertion of equivalence (X is Y). Since, however, the secondary subject is far from being identical with the first (the farther away the more striking the metaphor), the linguistic instruction to equate them can be obeyed only through interpretive activity. This consists of construing the secondary subject, the vehicle, as a set of meanings or an "implicative complex" (Black, 1979:28), and accommodating the topic to it by cancelling some elements of the complex and highlighting others (see, Cohen, 1979; Levin, 1979). The primary subject is refracted through the secondary complex, resulting in changes of its prior resonances, relations, and possibilities of meaning.

The cognitive functions of metaphor derive mainly from the fact that the amalgamation of primary and secondary subjects represents a possible world different from the conventional one in which they are distinct. The shock of a live metaphor is that of its prospective possibility rather than its literal impossibility. It is this that allows Black (1979:37) to argue that a metaphorical statement is capable of generating new knowledge, an argument convincingly substantiated by Schön (1979) through examples from technical invention and from policies on urban planning. What Schön calls generative metaphors do not, like similes, just trade on familiar equations—they create new ones. A metaphor takes the reader who follows it into a possible world where it can be literally true, which is to say into an unfamiliar cognitive framework: "metaphor bears information because it 'redescribes' reality" (Ricoeur, 1977:22). This is why metaphor has cognitive effects not merely stronger than those of metonymy but of a different order: it operates at the level of predicative statements and propositional sentences—the minimal units of discourse—whereas metonymy operates at the subdiscursive level of individual words.

One other property of metaphor worth stressing, because of its relevance to producing effects of reality as well as knowledge, is its synthesis of abstract and concrete representations of reality (that is, concepts and images). Langer (1948), approaching metaphorical thinking from an examination of visual perception, describes it as a peculiarly strong expression of "abstractive seeing" (p. 14) whereby concepts are abstracted from "the tumbling stream of impressions" (p. 117). Linguistically oriented theorists, however, tend to stress the role of metaphor in making abstract concepts concrete more than making concrete detail abstract. This follows from the typical linguistic structure of a metaphor, in which the primary subject is relatively abstract and the secondary one relatively concrete. Paivio (1979), a cognitive psychologist, argues that metaphors serve thought by pegging concrete nouns and images to abstract nouns, thus making them more comprehensible. Concreteness of the secondary subject, the vehicle, is said to be especially effective in promoting comprehension. The concretizing effects described by Paivio in terms of cognitive processing are described by rhetoricians in figures of speech such as personification, and referred to by literary theorists in terms of giving "visibility" and "perceptibility" to discourse (see, Moran, 1989:89–90; Ricoeur, 1977:149).

Metaphor is not, of course, the only or even the primary literary means of concretizing abstract concepts. Metonymy is especially important in this respect, which is to be expected from its grounding in experiential associations. Reddy (1979:300), for example, observes of metonymy that "when two entities are always found together in our experience, the name of one of them—usually the more concrete—will develop a new sense which refers to the other." So, pensioner comes to stand for older people. It must be stressed again, however, that metaphor has a special role in discourse because it concretizes at the level of predicative statements, the basic units of discourse, rather than individual words or phrases. The significance of metonymy for discourse analysis is shown once more to be an auxilliary one arising from its linkage to metaphor. Black (1979:31) helps to explicate the linkage in describing the cognitive dynamics of metaphor: "Every implication-complex supported by a metaphor's secondary subject . . . is a *model* of the ascriptions imputed to the primary subject: Every metaphor is the tip of a submerged model." We can say, then, that metaphors serve to articulate old and new, established and projected topics in a field of discourse. The role of metonyms is only to help draw out the latent models contained in metaphors: a subsidiary work of articulation and concretization.

I will proceed now to the metaphors of gerontology, using them to reveal further the discursive structure of the field.

METAPHORS OF THE AGED

I will begin with age and class. Considered as a metaphorical vehicle, social class is a set of predicative statements relating inequalities of life-chance and advantage to economic function, status valuation, and power position. Its linguistic paradigm or, using Saussure's term, associative field includes class stratification, class structure, class consciousness, class solidarity, class division, and class conflict. When age is inserted into this "implication-complex," or "model of ascriptions," a process of simple substitution yields a duplicate paradigm: age stratification, age structure, age consciousness, age solidarity, age division, and age conflict. The insertion is not a matter of saying that age can be correlated *with* class membership but that age *is* a kind of class membership. The duplicate paradigm projects newly possible knowledge objects and a methodical expansion of topics by means of analogical equivalence. It also certifies the substantive reality of the aged by making the category a standing reality that is as solid and thing-like as a social class. Emile Durkheim's injunction that the most fundamental rule of sociological observation is to "consider social facts as things" (Durkheim, 1938:14) can be regarded as a statement about the literary production of social facts and the kind of work metaphor, among other means, has to perform: a statement about the requirements of social science writing and reading rather than just those of research. Social phenomena must be made thing-like in the act of reading if social science discourse is to be possible. This is a major point to be demonstrated in the illustrative materials to follow. The illustrations themselves, however, concern the methodical expansion of topics and, thereby, the articulation of the master categories of gerontology across diverse details.

The amalgamation of age with class entails, as in all metaphorical equations, selective organization of the secondary complex. Given that class discourse has tended to selectively organize itself between a Marxian vocabulary of economically based division, exploitation, power, and conflict on the one hand, and a largely American social research vocabulary of culturally based status distinction on the other, it is not surprising to find the pattern repeated in class metaphors of the aged. Streib (1985) argues that the class identity of the elderly cannot be grounded in economic location because its members are typically outside the labor force. Consequently, he highlights status valuation, placing the aged in a status hierarchy of looking up and looking down rather than an economic arena of struggle between opponents:

> Generally, old age is not valued highly because it is associated widely with decline in physical attractiveness, vigor, health condition, sexual process, and perhaps some mental abilities. And most important from an actuarial basis, it is associated with the expectation of fewer years of life itself. In a fundamental sense, this is the consideration that makes the aged lose status. . . . The inescapable fact of human mortality forces all other aspects of ranking to fade when evaluated in relation to life itself . . . some persons who are most hostile to the aged as a category are those who are fearful of their own eventual decline and demise. They have not come to terms with their own mortality and shun contact with anyone who might remind them of their future condition. (Streib, 1985:341)

From this it is evident that some resonances of the status hierarchy variant of class metaphor are identical with the deficit accumulation metaphor of aging. They will be discussed further under that heading. Meanwhile, I want to fill in other features of this particular way of turning elderly people into a thought-object.

The lexicon of status differentiation includes terms to indicate seamless continuity up and down a class gradient. The terms upper, middle, and lower are only minimal indicators of the implicit model, which is that of a sliding scale. The model is fully explicated in refinements that have become standard in status research: upper–upper, middle–upper, lower–upper, upper–middle, middle–middle, lower–middle, upper–lower, middle–lower, lower–lower. Considered as an individual characteristic, old age, according to Streib and many others, pushes one down the social status scale. Gerontology, however, does not—and *cannot*—rest on old age as nothing but an individual characteristic: it is founded on aging and the aged as collective realities and collective concepts. This is why gerontological discourse goes beyond correlating age with other characteristics, and metaphorically turns the aged into a status group in its own right. The linguistic repercussions of this amalgamation help to articulate "the aged" (showing its nature in researchable predicates) and certify its substantive reality, thus paying a double discursive dividend. For example, just as each social status stratum splits into upper, middle, and lower, so the aged split, with seemingly natural credibility, into three categories. Streib (1985:351), following gerontological convention and in linguistic lockstep with status theory, describes them as the "young–old" (aged 55–65, usually working, at their peak in earning capacity and social recognition), the "middle–old" (aged 65–75, retired, with reduced income but in good health and active), and the "old–old" (aged 75 and over, including "those who are most frail, the sickest, the most isolated, and the most impoverished segment" of the older population, the "problem population" among the aged that metonymically devalues the category). Along the same lines of metaphorical equivalence, just as status theory posits multiple status indicators and the possibility of status inconsistents, so gerontologists talk of "age incongruents" who are chronologically in one age group but behave or function as if in another (Riley, 1985:391).

The political economic form of class metaphor construes the aged in a different lexicon. Here, classes are discrete actors, usually placed in antagonistic pairs or coalitional blocs, and articulated in terms such as victimization, conflict, class consciousness, and organized power. In this frame of reality construction, "the aged" refers to a systematically disadvantaged location within an economy of power relations. Hudson and Strate (1985:578–79) say: "The political economist sees the elderly as one social aggregation among many whose welfare is a function of a political system dominated by concentrated capital and class politics." Again, however, the discursive requirements of gerontology are such that it is not enough to say that elderly people's life chances are constrained by class location, elderly people themselves must be made into a distinctive collective reality. Hudson and Strate go on to say that "analysis of the aged and their problems" must be separated from "the same problems suffered by other have-not groups throughout society" (p. 579). The discursive requirement of making the aged a substantive entity dictates that the aged must *be* a class group. Linguistic repercussions and a resultant conceptual imaging of the aged follow from that identification. The aged is equated with the exploited working class in the secondary complex of the metaphor. Since, however, its disadvantaged position cannot in the face of retirement from work be directly attributed to workplace relations and the appropriation of surplus value, another matrix of class formation must be named. Estes et al. (1982), for example, welcome the stress of Poulantzas on political and ideological determina-

tions of class division because they "might be of importance in considering class relations among the aged *and of the aged with the non-aged*," but
"one would still wish for a definition of class which would take into
account the social and economic dynamics which directly involve *the
aged qua aged*" (Estes et al., 1982:158, emphases added). These authors go
on to formulate class conflict relations between the aged and the non-
aged in terms of the subordination of "aged subjects" to public and
private social welfare bureaucracies, substituting the administration of
"unilateral dependency" for ownership and control of the means of
economic production as the basis of class power, and substituting welfare bureaucrats for the bourgeoisie as the ruling class. Other gerontologists, sticking more closely to the aged qua aged, express conflict with
the nonaged in terms of working taxpayers versus nonworking consumers, specified here to generational conflict. Davis and van den Oever
(1981), for example, describe an intergenerational class struggle between
young and old over the distribution of wealth.

Finally, both variants of the 'age is class' metaphor make chronological
classification resonate with the connotations of class consciousness. The
case of political economic conflict is sufficiently obvious to require no
special comment. Streib (1985:350) draws an explicit anology between
class consciousness and age consciousness (an analogy being an explicated metaphor), and observes that "a shared victim status" (p. 355) is
the basis of "age solidarity and age consciousness" among the elderly.
The case of status differentiation deserves a little more attention since it
relates to the next metaphor to be considered: the aged is a minority
group.

Riley (1985:388–89), enunciating the status group notion of a collective
actor, says that the aged is a reality formed by "age integration" and
"age homophily." The former refers to historical and cultural "mutuality
of experiences, perceptions, and interests"; the latter refers to same age
interaction and communication in daily living. An age cohort is thus
turned into a life-style group defined by age-based practices of inclusion
and exclusion. This brings the aged into close linguistic proximity with
other life-style-defined entities. Cutler (1977:1024) observes that age
identification is comparable to class consciousness, partisan identification, sex identification, and ethnic identification: "to the degree to which
old people become aware of themselves as old, they may take on the
politically relevant characteristics of a minority group or subculture."
This points to a whole new complex of implications and another latent
model through which to articulate the aged: that of a minority group.

Kitzinger (1987:32), analyzing social scientific accounts of lesbians,
notes that the terminology of disease used to marginalize and control
this group has also been applied by psychologists to ethnic and other

minority group behavior deviant from the majority culture. In general, the diagnosis of mental illness is apt to be made of any life-style group representing a competing or contrary social reality and thus posing "a potential threat to the dominant social order" (p. 33). Pathology, disease, and mental disorder are, then, part of the semantic complex belonging to the term minority group, but only a part. Also to be included are protective and celebratory associations of the term: the minority group as persecuted victim and the minority group as countercultural hero. Kitzinger points, for example, to the interpretive trajectory of lesbians through the individual rights vocabulary of liberal humanism and the positive life-style vocabulary of gay affirmation.

Departure from a normal behavioral order is the basis of the implicative complex around "minority group," but the complex itself includes three wordways for construing minority departure: the vocabularies of pathology, civil rights protection, and countercultural celebration. All three have been used in gerontology to render the aged a legible and researchable object. In Chapter 2, reference was made to the geriatric concept of old age as a progressive disease. The concept resonates obliquely in the metaphor of deficit accumulation, to be discussed later in this chapter. At the opposite valuational extreme—though within the same metaphor complex—are celebrations of golden oldies, prime timers, gray is beautiful, and Gray Panther power. The last two lexical items, it should be noted, are metonymic extensions of black minority group affirmation, providing linguistic evidence in support of our line of argument.

Regarding minority persecution and protection, the most important discipline concept coined from this part of the complex is ageism. It was developed by straightforward linguistic transfers: from racial discrimination to age discrimination, from racial prejudice to age prejudice, from racism to ageism: "a process of systematic stereotyping of and discrimination against people because they are old, just as racism and sexism accomplish this with skin color and gender" (Butler, 1969:244). These linguistic transfers, I would add, while straightforward in the local language practices of gerontology, allowing ageism to become in gerontology a standard unit of discursive exchange, have not been straightforward in the languages of law and legislation. Eglit (1985) points out that in the United States the legal concept of a "suspect" classification— meaning one so burdened with systematic disadvantage, persistent inequality, or powerlessness as to require special protection in the majoritarian political process—has been applied to race and ethnicity but not, or not consistently, to age. In the legal field of reality construction, age lines are weak classifiers and dubious—because arguably rational— criteria of discrimination. Thus a Supreme Court decision in favor of the

Massachusetts Board of Retirement (Massachusetts Board of Retirement
v. Murgia, 1976) on the issue of compulsory retirement for police officers
at age 50 said that old age does not define a "discrete and insular group"
because everyone goes into it. Legislation aimed against ageism such as
the Age Discrimination Act (1975) and the Age Discrimination in Employment Act (1978) has stumbled across the same lack of determinacy:

> At least in the areas of racism and sexism, the victims are fairly clearly
> identifiable: one is either black or not; one is either a woman or not. In
> contrast, age, the trigger for discrimination in the context of ageism, is a
> characteristic that all possess to a greater or lesser degree. (Eglit, 1985:542)

The questionable recognizability of age lines is also evident in jury
selection. Juries are required to represent a fair cross section of the
community. The courts have, however, consistently rejected age group
representation on the grounds that age groups are neither "distinctive"
nor "cognizable" (Eglit, 1985:538). These would be startling and dismay-
ing claims if transposed to gerontology, where the distinctiveness and
cognizability of age groups are indispensable conditions of inquiry. The
point I would make, however, is not that gerontology is built on sand
but that the solidity and certainty of thought-objects are in every discipline internally conferred by local language practices and never externally granted by objective existence. Also, that there is never an automatic translation of the latent model of reality contained in a metaphor
complex into an accepted manifest model: the former has to be discursively worked up into the latter, and the outcome is not foregone. This is
evident in the case of gerontology and the minority group metaphor.
The descriptive formulations of aging and the aged in gerontology and
the articulation of gerontological topics, issues, and conjectures all testi-
fy to acceptance of the metaphor and its latent model. At the level of
overt theorizing, however, there is disagreement.

Streib (1965) asks: "Are the aged a minority group?" Here and elsewhere (Streib 1985), he argues that they are not. Elderly people do not
share "a distinct and separate culture" (1985:352) and membership is
something that comes to everyone rather than being exclusive or perma-
nent. Others are less sure. Drake (1958) hesitates to call the aged a full
minority group, as argued by Barron (1953), because it has no unique
history, language, or culture; nonetheless, it is stereotyped by the majority, does suffer collective discrimination, and does display self-conscious
sensitivity and defensiveness, so he is willing to call it a "quasi-minority
group." Others, like Rose (1965), see the development of a subculture of
the aged based on demographic volume, selective interaction, housing
segregation, common policy interests, and the like. I do not wish to
pursue these shades of opinion; my point is that the minority group

metaphor inscribes a clear topical agenda in the field, allowing indeed for the founding of a distinct subarea called ethnogerontology, and this shows the field to be informed by the metaphor regardless of manifest theoretical endorsement.

METAPHORS OF AGING

Deficit Accumulation

The metaphor of aging as deficit accumulation was mentioned in connection with the aged as a status group. Also it articulates the geriatric model of aging as a progressive disease with one of the cultural foundations of gerontology described in Chapter 2: the deviancy of old age from core values of our social–moral order.

Explicit references to deficit accumulation are mainly clustered in biological and psychological accounts of aging. Here the highlighted features of aging are progressive losses of physiological, sensory, and cognitive functioning. These are, however, related metonymically to losses of social functioning, providing a linguistic matrix for theoretical models of status loss, role loss, and loss of positive social identity. For example, Rosow (1985) identifies old age with "social loss" (p. 69) and deploys a deficit accumulation vocabulary of "role emptying," "shrinkage within roles," and decrement of "vital functions" (pp. 70–71 passim) to represent the process of becoming old. The vocabulary represents common linguistic recipes of aging—take care of yourself, keep active, don't overdo it, find a hobby—as platitudes, the emptiness of which "simply documents the empty social role of the aged, the general irreversibility of their losses, and their ultimate solitude in meeting their existential declines" (Rosow, 1985:72).

These words bring out a crucial element of the secondary complex of the metaphor: the fatalism associated with cumulative deficits. It is this that leads Eisdorfer and Cohen (1980) to urge a distinction between "primary aging" (deficits occurring as a direct function of biological aging) and "secondary aging" (those occurring as an indirect function of time through a higher probability of experiencing accidents, stresses, diseases, and so on, the longer one lives)—a distinction, I would say, between the biological and statistical fates of aging. It is this also that underlies their interesting declaration that the concept of deficit is not only a description and explanation of age-related changes in behavior, but "a nihilistic metaphor" (Eisdorfer and Cohen, 1980:60). By this they mean that the idea of inevitable, irreversible losses of function annhilates therapeutic hope and positive personal expectations. From the standpoint of language analysis, something else needs to be added. Deficit accumulation is an implicative complex belonging to bookkeeping. Also belonging to the complex is the final balance, the now colloquial "bottom line." The bottom line of aging is death, and death is a topic of special significance not only for gerontology but for discourse as such.

The significance of death as a topic for gerontology is textually evident in the existence of a sub area, thanatology, specially devoted to it, and in stock pedagogical subjects of the field: stages of death, euthanasia, palliative care, mourning and grief, death settings, and the hospice movement. Its significance for discourse as such requires us to step back into language theory.

All discourse is informed by a desire for rational articulation in the face of a gap or dissonance between what we can say and what we want to say, more exactly, between logical means of representation and other figurations or imprints of experience. Death is something about which, above all other topics, consciously mortal beings desire rational representation. Yet it is a topic that language theorists declare to be peculiarly resistant to representation, a signified so totally removed from signifiers that it represents a virtual end of rational representation itself. Eco (1976:66) advances the familiar semiotic view that sign-vehicles (for example, the word *death*) are circulated "in place of things," implying that things are endlessly deferred in language. He adds that the only thing that cannot be thus "semioticized" is death, once it has occurred. The word *death* in linguistic use refers to a moment before the absolute end and is, therefore, still lodged in a cultural order of experience. The word stands in place of the thing that would end rational representation, and so defers that end. Discursive multiplication of death as a cultural unit endlessly postpones the only thing that can silence discourse.

Since, in our cultural order, old people are symbolic figurations and living icons of death, it is inevitable that the study of aging should turn, through metonymic connection, to dying and that the topic should loom large in gerontology. The deficit accumulation metaphor highlights the topic with particular clarity but, as we shall see, every metaphor of aging leads representation in the same direction.

I would add one more comment on the dialectic of articulation and deferral evident in gerontological occupancy of what is called death. The dialectic receives added strength and subtlety from a cultural order wanting to deny death and its virtual defeat of rational representation. The denial of death, the absolute end, the truly bottom line, is performed in gerontology through a profuse cultivation of *death*, the cultural unit: a striking example of the cunning of language. Back and Baade (1966:302) say: "the predominant attitude of American society toward death is the complete denial of its presence and concomitantly a complete discontinuity of the dead with the living." In American gerontology a compensatory reversal is evident. Death, in its moments and settings of social occurrence, is expressly affirmed and the living are, through, for example, finely graded stage theories of dying (Kubler-Ross, 1969), made continuous with the virtually dead. Correlative with a cultural denial of death, the absolute end, is a discursive circulation of *death* the cultural unit. The desires for denial and rational representation of the same thing are thus met in a single discursive trajectory.

The same dialectic and trajectory help make sense of the puzzling prominence of the term frailty in gerontology. Frailty is a metonymic associate of dying and thus belongs both to the discursive cultivation of death (its "semioticization" and theorization), and to deferral of death–deferral both of the cultural unit (since it stands metonymically in place of the word death) and of the absolute end (since *death* and all its linguistic surrogates stand in place of the unnamable thing). *Frailty* thus fuses the opposite desires of denial and representation in a way continuous with *death*, and with an extra metonymic twist. It can, for this reason, be called an overdetermined concept in gerontological usage. It has a special affinity with deficit accumulation—though having a much wider circulation—because it designates that segment of the aged—sometimes called "the very old–old" (Loeb and Borgatta, 1980:196)—on the borderline with death, in which is concentrated physical, mental, and social loss. Beyond the very old–old and their multiple deficits lies the continuous gradient to death articulated in thanatology.

Life Cycle, Passage, Convoy, and Journey

These four metaphors of aging, although linguistically close to each other, represent distinct latent models of becoming old. The differences can be described in terms of determinism vs. voluntarism, familiar from a broader vocabulary the human sciences use to describe methodological options. The life cycle model carries biological connotations of inevitability and causal predetermination that are in distinct contrast to the voluntaristic, open discovery connotations of a journey. Passage and convoy are intermediate models in terms of this contrast. The former is closer to causal determinism in that it highlights individual movement through societally predetermined channels and past societally given stage markers; the latter is closer to voluntarism in that it highlights typical companions and typical changes of companion in the journey of aging.

The determinism–voluntarism distinction is, in turn, an expression of the pull between scientistic and humanistic tendencies that characterizes all human science. In gerontology one can see it played out through the contributory disciplines of the field. Scientistic determinism is especially strong in biological, biomedical, and psychological constructs of becoming old. Philibert's (1982) critique of the scientistic fallacy in gerontology, the mistaken yearning to capture the reality of aging in experimental observation and objective laws, points especially to its grounding in studies of cells, tissues, muscular power, heart activity, memory, verbal fluidity, and the like: a search for laws of decline following a scientistic trajectory of "genetic, biochemical, physiological, psychological" studies leading, via demography, into the social sciences (Philibert, 1982:307). The deterministic continuity between biological and psychological models of aging is illustrated in Neugarten's (1981) account of developmental processes in the "psychology of the life cycle" (p. 208). These are of two general kinds: "processes that are biologically programmed and inherent in the organism," and emergent processes of adaptation through which "the organism is irreversibly changed or transformed by interaction with the environment" (Neugarten, 1981:209). Such models, hooked to the notion of deficit accumulation, were no doubt the occasion for the protest by the Gray Panthers, cited by Estes (1979:226), that gerontology reinforces views of older people "as stuck in an inevitable chronological destiny of decay and deterioration."

The opposite kind of model, voluntaristic humanism, is carried into gerontology mostly by its historical and anthropological tributaries. Both, as a matter of approach, seek to recreate *experiences* of aging and thus engage linguistically in intersubjective understanding as well as objective representation. Achenbaum (1985:130) claims that historians have been the main contributors to humanistic research in gerontology: "methodologically . . . history serves as a bridge between the social sciences and the humanities." Comparably, Van Tassel and Stearns (1986:xix) observe that historians of old age "are united by a lively sympathy for the objects of their study" and "in their own way . . . contribute also to the essential battle against some of the routinizing tendencies of a bureaucratic society." The models of aging supplied to gerontology by its contributory disciplines thus mark political as well as methodological differences in the field.

If scientific determinism and humanistic voluntarism are poles of conceptual variation in models of aging, then not only explicit discipline models but latent metaphor models can be ranged between them, and in a roughly parallel order. The life cycle metaphor is basically psychobiological whereas passage, convoy, and journey are metaphors belonging more to anthropology and history; sociology characteristically stretches between the poles. My present purpose, however, is to examine the metaphors rather than the discursive roles played in gerontology by associated disciplines. In this connection, the life cycle metaphor projects a distinct conceptual image of becoming old, an image cast in advance of deliberate thought, two features of which are especially significant for shaping discourse. One is the placement of the aging individual in the grammatical position of an object to which events happen, or of a reactor to events, rather than being an active subject, author, or initiator of events. The other feature is the stratified division of the self into a biological substructure, the base of aging events, and a personal, sociocultural superstructure added reactively over time. The conceptual effect is to partition individuals into a universal common denominator and an emergent, contingent identity, the former having causal priority over the latter.

These features can be recovered from the gerontological concept of aging clock theory (Harris, 1988:17), proposing that aging is timed by a mechanism in the hypothalamus, and the broader distinction made between biological and social clocks. Researchers refer to all neural and endocrine regulators of aging as "pacemakers" (Harris, 1988:132). Neugarten (1981:215), representing a causal law psychology and sociology of aging, observes that biology is not "the sufficient pacemaker of personality change" and account must also be taken of "the social clock that is superimposed over the biological clock in establishing rhythms of stability and change." Strehler (1977) describes the imperatives of the biological clock as intrinsic and determinate processes of aging, contrasting these with ancillary processes arising from culture, society, habits, and the environment.

In contrast to the life cycle metaphor of aging, where sociobiological events happen to people according to externally set mechanisms, the metaphors of passage and journey project active individuals going through events. Events now have the status of a landscape to be individually traversed, and of a timetable to be consulted en route rather than a deterministic schedule of universal stages. Hagestad and Neugarten (1985), contributing to the second edition of Binstock and Shanas' *Handbook of Aging and the Social Sciences*, speak of a shift in the field, since the 1976 first edition, from a life cycle to a life course orientation. The latter, conveyed in metaphors of passage, convoy, and journey, focuses on "pathways along an age-differentiated, socially created sequence of transitions" (Hagestad and Neugarten, 1985:36). These are said to provide "roadmaps of human lives" (p. 35) and a means for individuals to find direction and make sense of "the passage of individual life time" (p. 36). There are "rites of passage," "social ceasings and becomings," and "points in life" that are "punctuations of the life line" (p. 37). They give legible coherence, both societally and subjectively, to the time between birth and death. Keith (1985:253) notes that in modern old age where "exit signs" are numerous and entry signs few or poorly posted, individuals do significatory things like plunging into volunteer work and going on extended travel—in effect supplying their own punctuation to make up for lack of societal markers of meaningful period and transition. That actual travel should become a marker of the life journey is a compression of the primary into the secondary subject of the metaphor, an imitation or forgery of a literal statement that thereby confirms its metaphorical status.

The generative capacity of the passage and journey metaphors to articulate topics around aging is already evident in the preceding materials. Further documentation is provided by Hagestad and Neugarten (1985). Pathways can be identified in terms of role transitions. Role transitions can be specified in terms of timing, spacing (the length of time between transitions, say between starting work and getting married), sequence, and duration (the average length of time it takes a cohort to complete a given transition). Age careers can be compared between individuals, groups, and societies. It is possible to study "transition domino effects" (p. 47)—how, say, adolescent parenthood triggers early exit from school, the effects of on-time and off-time transitions on social competence and personality development, the relative salience of different tracks and pathways for different social groups, the intersection of pathways among consociates, "pictures of individuals' life progress through key transition roadmarkers" (p. 54), and "cohort transition snapshots" (p. 54).

The convoy metaphor of aging yields further articulation and wider occupancy of the virtual subject matter designated by aging and the aged, by focusing on kinship networks, significant others, and social relationships:

> The term Convoy of social support is used to describe the dynamic concept of social networks over the life course . . . a variety of interpersonal relationships become the bases for the support Convoy. . . . At different points in the life course, members of the Convoy may be lost either through death or less radical changes. At the same time, as the individual matures, experiencing different life events and transitions, new Convoy members are added. (Antonucci, 1985:97)

Topics such as convoy size, connectedness, stability, complexity, functioning, and adequacy emerge readily from the metaphor, and fit readily with the conceptual agendas of passage and journey.

I would make only one other observation on life course metaphors. Although they predominantly imply voluntaristic humanism—most clearly in the metaphor of journeying with its implications of adventure and discovery, reminiscent of T. S. Eliot's line in "East Coker" (*Four*

Quartets): "Old men ought to be explorers"—they can be given a deterministic cast and thus brought close to the life cycle complex. This is apparent in accounts of aging pitched at the collective rather than individual level of analysis. Here the journeying subject is a group or category—most commonly, a cohort—passing through preset entry and exit points in an almost predestined way. For example, Riley (1985:392) describes how individual aging and cohort flow "operate in tandem to sort people into age strata and to channel people through the age-graded roles." As individuals age biologically and psychologically "they also move diagonally up through the age strata" (p. 392), passing through socially scheduled role transitions in more or less orderly patterns. Hagestad and Neugarten (1985:41) refer to age norms of permission, proscription, and prescription governing "role entries and exits." They add that "much of the research that has been labeled life course analysis does not analyze lives. Rather it presents statistical histories of birth cohorts" (p. 45). Where journeying describes an ineluctable passage through collectively set transition points according to a collectively dictated timetable, it draws linguistically and conceptually close to life cycle propulsion through predefined stages. Life course metaphors encourage but do not guarantee a voluntaristic, humanistic representation of aging.

NARRATIVITY AND ARTICULATION

I wish to recall the argument made in Chapter 1 that narration is essential to writing human science. Within the present topic of how gerontology occupies its field, the argument means that the appropriation process must exploit narrativity in the materials being appropriated in order to produce readably *human* and *social* science. A distorted glimpse of the argument is to be found in some observations by Stern (1990) on historiography. Historians, by virtue of their discipline, must *interpret the significance* of happenings in time, not merely *describe* them. They must distinguish between natural and nonnatural events and focus on the latter. The indispensable literary means of doing so is story telling: "Accounts of non-natural events tell us what a purposeful agent did or brought about. . . . Only in narrative can a non-natural event's significance—in a descriptive or evaluative sense of this word—become clear" (Stern, 1990:556, 557).

I call this a distorted glimpse of what I wish to argue, for two reasons. First, Stern obscures the constitutive role of narration in *producing* human science because he locates the natural–nonnatural distinction in events themselves rather than in how they are represented. If an earthquake is represented as the grumbling of an angry earth spirit it *is* a nonnatural event, whereas in a seismological description it *is* a natural event. It is the mode of representation that makes an event natural or nonnatural, not some inherent character or essence of the event itself. My argument is, then, that a human science, to be such, must include literary means of making its materials into nonnatural events, and that narrative is in this respect indispensable. The second reason for calling Stern's observations a distorted glimpse is that he lacks a clear concept of narrative (Fain, 1990:571). I will try to avoid that criticism by offering, briefly, a concept of narrative and narrativity drawn from semiotics and literary theory.[1]

Narratives in the ordinary sense—that is, the sense culturally familiar to us—recount events in time happening to and stemming from human or human-like actors. The two most salient features identifying a narrative are temporal sequence and anthropomorphic figures invested with thought, will, and feeling. For semiotics these are points of departure. Semiotic analysis moves simultaneously from temporal sequence to structural correlation (from diachrony to synchrony), and from surface representations to underlying systems of meaning (from semantic content to semiological grammar). Anticipations of this line of analysis can be found in Russian Formalism (see Jameson, 1972:43–98 for a useful overview). Especially important here is Propp's (1968) morphological study of Russian folk tales. Diverse story lines are reduced to abstract episodic units (e.g., injury → retribution, lack → acquisition), and diverse characters to standard figures (hero, villain, traitor, donor, magical agent). Every actual folk tale is shown to be a possibility drawn from 31 functional units according to law-like regularities of selection and combination.

In contemporary semiotics the most rigorous and far-reaching formulations along these lines are the writings of Greimas (1987:Chs. 4–8; 1989a–d) on narrative grammar. As in all grammatical analysis, there is a strong distinction in Greimas's model between realized utterances and the structural sources or latent possibilities of meaningful utterance. Directly relevant for my concern to describe how the disciplinary field of gerontology articulates a subject matter is the intended scope of the model. It applies not only to tales, stories, myths, and nonliterary as well as literary narratives, but to all enunciations of meaning: "the generation of meaning . . . is relayed . . . by narrative structures and it is these that produce meaningful discourse articulated in utterances" (Greimas, 1987:65).

---

[1] Two helpful resources here are a special issue of *New Literary History*, Spring 1989 on Greimassian semiotics, and a special issue of *Critical Inquiry*, Autumn 1980, on narrative.

At the deepest level of narrative structure is the semiotic square (see Figure 1 and accompanying discussion): a latent arrangement of contrary, contradictory, and implicative relations that allows, and indeed pushes, a significatory unit into performative utterance. Since narratives articulate possibilities of meaning built into the semiotic square of signification, all materials having this structure may be said to possess narrativity. The materials of gerontology, as we have seen, have a semiotic structure by virtue of being representations of old age. Like any human science, therefore, gerontology exploits a narrativity already built into its subject matter. The interest of the model is in helping to specify how this is done in the surface utterances of a particular field of study.

From this standpoint, the strategically crucial part of narrative grammar is that which deals with actions of language. An utterance is an action whereby a predicate is modified by a subject. A narrative, we might say, is a linguistic action whereby an initial state of affairs is modified so as to turn into another. Modifications are associated linguistically with modal verbs, so Greimas calls this part of narrative grammar the theory of modalities (Greimas, 1987:Ch. 7). It should be understood, however, that even though a description of the modalities must give them a semantic interpretation, they are intended—like all other elements of the grammar—to be syntactic patterns open to the most varied semantic content in actual utterances. They are formal structures of linguistic action that, in substantive materials, allow for the representation of psychological and social actions. Narrative representations of actions are carried and sustained by effectively present actions of the linguistic medium. Modalities refer to the latter.

Greimas reasons that if an act is some kind of "making to be," then an act of (and in) language must rest on two kinds of predicates: doing and being. So there are two possible forms of elementary utterances: utterances of doing and utterances of state or condition. Utterances of state locate a grammatical subject (an actant) in relation to an object or situation of value. (The basic possibilities are conjunction, disjunction, nonconjunction, and nondisjunction.) Utterances of doing express transformation from one state to another. Narratives bring together predicates of being and doing in various patterns of mutual modification. The basic patterns specified by the theory of modalities are wanting-(to-do, to-be), having-to-(do or be), being-able-(to-do or to-be), knowing-how-to-(do or be), and causing-to-(do or be). This seemingly sparse set of meaning spaces is greatly elaborated by two theoretical considerations. First, the logic of the semiotic square demands that each term be elaborated into a four-fold structure. For example:

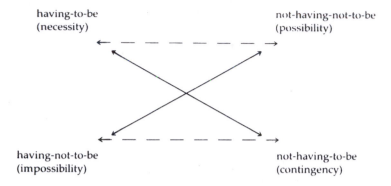

having-to-be
(necessity)

not-having-not-to-be
(possibility)

having-not-to-be
(impossibility)

not-having-to-be
(contingency)

Just as narratives of the transformation of necessity into contingency and possibility can be spun from this particular square, so narratives of the transformation of desire into possession, obedience into resistance, knowledge into ignorance, certainty into wisdom, and capacity into incapacity can be spun from the semiotic squares of the other modalities.

The second theoretical consideration is that the modal structures can be combined in pairs so that one semiotic square is superimposed on another. For example, having-to-be can be superimposed on wanting-to-be. The extra twist here is that the two squares can be in a compatible alignment (where having-to is aligned with wanting-to in the first corner of the joint square), or in an incompatible alignment (where having-to is aligned either with not-wanting-to-be or actively wanting-not-to-be). An actual narrative might, then, rotate two superimposed squares through possible combinations of compatibility and incompatibility. The point is, however, that every actual narrative whatsoever articulates possibilities of linguistic action granted by these underlying syntactic structures. This applies, therefore, to the narratives of gerontology about aging and the collective actant of aging: the aged. They trade on a semiotic narrativity built into their materials.

To return the discussion to the surface narratives of gerontology, we must make central a feature basic to the story design of narratives but deliberately suspended in structural and grammatical analysis: this is temporality, the placement of actions in a temporal sequence. Greimas's narrative grammar does not exclude temporality. It is allowed for in the construction of the semiotic square that *begins*, in the *first* corner, with a significatory element, and then expands through operations of active negation and passive contradiction into the second, third, and fourth corners. Temporality is also allowed for in the idea that modalities are ranged from those that initially institute a subject (the "virtualizing" modalities of wanting and having-to), through those that qualify the subject in terms of competence (the "actualizing" modalities of being-able and knowing-how), to the "realizing" modality of causing-to-be, where another state appears. These allowances for temporality are still, however, too deeply layered and abstract to capture the temporality of story lines. For this we need narrower and more direct concepts.

Ricoeur (1980) has turned his attention to precisely this problem and uses the concept of plot to help solve it:

> By plot I mean the intelligible whole that governs a succession of events in any story. . . . A story is *made out of* events to the extent that plot *makes* events *into* a story. The plot, therefore, places us at the crossing point of temporality and narrativity. (Ricoeur, 1980:171)

In a field of discourse, narratives develop around the governing concepts (or what I have called legisigns) of the field. Two kinds of plots can be distinguished. Some narratives conceptually unfold the denotative and connotative meanings of a legisign. These can be called *theory plots*. Other narratives locate a legisign within an overview of the field it governs, telling of the importance of the phenomenon it names and certifying its discursive centrality for the discipline concerned. These can be called *field plots*. Both are crucial in articulating a subject matter.

In gerontology, the main theory plots of aging have been disengagement theory, activity theory, and developmental (or continuity) theory. (Other plots have emerged from criticisms at the margin of gerontology, especially the political economy approach, but I will defer discussion of these to the concluding chapter.) The plots are different as theories, being in this respect rival competitors, but as narratives they have much in common. Each of them is a normalizing narrative inscribed on and against cultural representations of aging as a deviance (gradual and/or catastrophic) from ordinary, canonical membership of society. (See Chapter 2 for value definitions of canonical membership.) Each one is also a good news narrative inscribed on and against cultural representations of gloom and despair in old age. Each in its own way transforms becoming old from something negative to something positive. The cogency of all three narratives depends, therefore, on the textual presence of negative cultural representations of aging. Without them the narratives would have no point, and the theories corresponding to them would degenerate into socially empty formalities.

One other common feature arises from the requirements of narration as such. Danto (1965:236–237) says that a narrative is an interpretive explanation of how one state of affairs turns, over time, into another. What makes the account a narrative, however, is the introduction of a new element—a means, agency or mediator—not present (or at least only latently so) in the initial state. All three gerontological plots of aging rest, therefore, on the introduction of novelty and contingency into apparently ineluctable necessity. In terms of content, the role of ineluctable necessity is played in gerontology by biological aging: loss of bone mass, stiffening blood vessels, decrease in reaction time, and so on: "True aging is *intrinsic* to the organism. A person cannot change or manipulate the rate of this process" (Novak, 1988:78). Since narrative requires some openness of outcome, there can be no narrative of purely biological aging. It must be overlaid and punctuated with contingencies of individual life-style, personal attitudes, societal definitions, institutional arrangements, and deliberate intervention. It is through such breaches of necessity that narratological predicates (the syntactic modalities of narrative described by Greimas) can be inserted. Conversely, the insertion of such predicates breaches necessity and makes room for human (or anthropomorphic) actors. The theory plots of gerontology vary in their selection and combination of predicates from the pool of modalities; consequently, they vary in the way actors are formulated. They also vary in their distributions of knowledge and competence between actors, a point that requires further explanation.

In gerontology, the most obviously significant actor is the aged. According to Greimassian theory, actors are narratively formulated by (1) being invested with modalities of performance, competence, and being, and (2) being assigned to an actant role. Greimas (1987:107) observes that a single actor can combine more than one actant position, or, conversely, one actant can be narratively incarnated by several actors. The basic actant positions are subject, object, sender, receiver, helper, opponent, enunciator, and enunciatee (that is, listener or reader). The last pair are distinct because they belong to the axis of communication rather than the plane of content. They are "actants of communication" rather than "actants of narration" (Greimas and Courtés, 1989:568). They are of primary importance in a field of discourse, where content is a knowledge object transmitted from enunciator to reader, and especially in gerontology with its strong activist, interventionist orientation. Due to its constitution, gerontology must formulate *itself* in actantial terms, both in the enunciator position and in its narratives of aging. Gerontology articulates itself in articulating its subject matter. In narratively formulating the aged, gerontologists narratively formulate themselves and their field.

This idea can be given a more specific expression. The gerontologist, whether speaking critically, humanistically, or operating behind the third person, passive construction style of natural science, is giving voice to a narrative subject: the aged. In accordance with the fiduciary contract of all human science, the gerontologist gives voice by telling the truth of the subject's doing and being to someone who might not know.

From the standpoint of distinguishing between theory plots, a crucial consideration is the amount of knowledge and competence invested by predicates of aging in the aged. This determines how much room and call there is for the narrative operator to speak for the narrative subject. At issue here is the scope and power of the actant position open to gerontology. In comparing theory plots, the position will be seen to depend on the knowledge and competence predicated of the aged by the modalities used to represent aging.

Disengagement theory, first sketched by Cumming et al. (1960) and elaborated by Cumming and Henry (1961), portrays aging through predicates of role loss and reduced social participation: "The life space of an individual decreases with age, in that he or she interacts with a narrower variety of role partners and spends a smaller proportion of his or her time in interaction" (Wershow, 1981:78). This not merely a reduction in the amount of social participation, however, but also a change in form. Obligatory, instrumental roles are progressively shed, leaving a purer residue of voluntary, expressive roles: "freedom from obligation replaces the constraint of being needed in an interlocking system of divided tasks. The fully engaged man is, in essence, bound; the disengaged man is free—if he has resources and health enough to allow him to exercize that freedom" (Cumming [1963], 1981:44). To the predicates of role loss and shrinkage of social participation must be added predicates of enhanced choice and subjective preference.

Also to be added, finally, are predicates of knowledge and wisdom. The disengagement process proceeds "as if agreed upon by all concerned" (Cumming [1963], 1981:46). The aging individual gains freedom while others (society) benefit from a minimization of disruption when the individual dies. Awareness of death is, in fact, the agency of mediation between the states of engagement and disengagement. Disengagement begins in middle age and is initiated by "an urgent new perception of the inevitability of death" (Cumming [1963], 1981:43). The turning point of the narrative resides in the narrative subject and consists of an acknowledgment of what has to be.

In terms of the basic modalities of narrative, disengagement theory combines having-to, wanting-to, and knowing-how-to in a compatible alignment: what the narrative subject has to do is also what the subject wants and knows how to do.

These observations allow us to explain the oddly central yet negative place of disengagement theory in gerontology. To do so it must be assumed that a human and social science must want to do things with words over and above establishing and explaining facts. By its character it must also want to move minds to action and make itself an effective actor in human affairs. This is especially true of gerontology with its orientation to policy intervention and practical application, but would apply to any recognizably human and social science. Thus to Weber's two criteria of adequacy at the level of causality and adequacy at the level of subjective meaning (Weber, 1978:11–12), we need also judge the adequacy of theories at the level of communicative action, which is to say, at the level of rhetoric and narrative effect.

Disengagement theory has been resisted in gerontology more strenuously than its causal or interpretive inadequacies can account for, and over a longer period than makes sense if these inadequacies are so blatant. As Estes (1978:43) comments: "the disengagement model has been more used as a 'strawman' than as a basis for intensive empirical examination." Its inadequacies (which fit it so well to be a "strawman") are to be found, I would argue, at the level of communicative action. Considered as a plot, disengagement theory has two shortcomings that make it unacceptable in the field.

First, disengagement theory is a minimalist narrative because aging is made close to being a predestined unfolding of natural events rather than a contingent emergence of nonnatural events (recalling Stern's distinction cited previously). Consequently, there is not much of an interpretive story to tell and the enunciator (the gerontology writer) is reduced to something more like a recorder and onlooker of natural sequences than a participant in communicative action: "As proposed by Cumming and Henry, the theory argues that the older person naturally or inevitably withdraws his or her emotional and actual involvement. . . . The disengagement process was considered to be natural or inherent because of the inevitability of death and the onset of physiological inabilities" (Cutler, 1977:1015). It is true that Cumming ([1963], 1981) "revisited" the theory and introduced a measure of contingency, hence of narrativity, through a distinction between "impinging" and "selector" temperaments that affect modes of withdrawal. The temperaments themselves, however, are said to be innate dispositions so there is only a small increment in narrativity and still no active place of intervention for gerontology.

The second narratological failing of disengagement theory is that the central narrative subject, the aged, is so fully invested with all the virtualizing and performative capacities needed to change the initial state into the end state that there is little scope for other actors. Certainly there is nothing of note for gerontology to do except, as indicated previously, to take notes and record events: "At the societal level, the theory discounts attempts to intervene in the aging process" (Estes, 1978:43).

Activity theory also depicts aging as a transition from societally compelled activity to a happy individual end, but the collective actant of the change is differently composed. The compositional predicates of the aged are now those of increased and qualitatively enhanced engagement with others rather than withdrawal and reduction. According to Harris's *Dictionary of Gerontology*: "activity theory stresses a continuation of role performances and asserts that the more active older persons are, the higher their life satisfaction and morale . . . older persons who age optimally are those who find substitutes for the activities and roles that they are forced to relinquish" (Harris, 1988:3). The plot can be complicated by questions of quality versus quantity of interaction, what kinds of activity are most conducive to high morale, and whether solitary activities like reading and watching television count for much (Lemon et al. [1972], 1981), but the outline is clear.

A significant extension of the activity narrative is the personal growth model. Kalish (1981) criticizes "geriactivist" theory for placing often impossibly high expectations on elderly people. In terms of Erikson's stages of adulthood, so influential in the social psychology of aging (see the review in Novak, 1988:128–133), the aging individual can choose intimacy over isolation, generativity over stagnation, and ego integrity over despair.

The extension is analytically significant because it points up the high degree of contingency built into activity theory. This not only invests the aged with several narratory degrees of freedom (hence, complex narrativity) but provides a major actant position for gerontology to occupy: that of a helper. The latter point is of great importance since it helps to explain why activity theory, in spite of low empirical confirmation (something admitted even by its advocates, for example, Lemon et al. [1972], 1981:31), is so popular in the field. Its appeal at the level of communicative action ensures it a positive reception completely independent of empirical adequacy. This way of articulating the subject matter of gerontology makes gerontology, in turn, a crucial narrative subject. To see how, and the kind of actant provided for, it is helpful to move down to the level of narrative modalities. It is in their selection and combination, particularly in dissonant combinations, that activity theory makes narrative room for gerontology and its narrators.

Without even attempting a technical narratological analysis, it can be seen that the plot first inscribes people in having-to-do situations of work, parenting and so on, which are compatibly combined with wanting-to, knowing-how-to, and being-able-to-do. Relinquishment, as a compulsory function of aging, turns have-to-do into either its contrary form (having-not-to-do) or its contradictory form (not-having-to-do). In either event dissonances are introduced with wanting-to, knowing-how-to, and being-able-to-do. The dissonances are resolved, in the plot of activity theory, by (1) continuing as many activities as possible (taking advantage of the optionality in not-having-to-do situations and separating these clearly from prohibitive having-not-to-do rules), and (2) finding substitutes for no longer possible activities (that is, wanting-to and knowing-how-to-do whatever is permitted). Resolution of dissonance is threatened, however, by a major opponent: misperception. Options and permissions can be mistaken for prohibitions, and the positive terms of wanting-to, knowing-how-to, and being-able-to-do can be turned into their negatives, yielding states of false closure and false necessity. The culprit here consists of cultural stereotypes of passive, frail, dependent old age. The helper role opened up for gerontology is that of exposing and reversing false consciousness: an exhortatory, tuitionary, and interventionist role. Kalish (1981:241) says: "*We can communicate to* older persons that *we have faith* in their abilities, that *we recognize* that they are capable of making decisions (even those decisions that we assume, perhaps correctly, will turn out wrong), that *we respect* their ownership of their own bodies and time and lives. In brief, *we can communicate* a Success Model instead of the Failure Models" (emphases added). Small wonder then that activity theory, regardless of empirical adequacy, is such a favored narrative in gerontology and so much more "congenial to gerontologists" (Estes, 1978:43) than disengagement theory. The latter way of articulating aging has the effect of disengaging gerontology from the scene of narration, thus contradicting a founding interest of the field in causing old age to be better.

Continuity theory, as the name implies, is a narrative of steady change over biological and biographical aging. It emphasizes the stability of personal identity against changes of role and circumstance, denying, for example, that work is such a crucial, indispensible source of identity that retirement must be a critical episode for individuals. Atchley ([1971], 1981) argues that our cultural means of self-definition include an ethic of leisure as well as a work ethic, and that retirement is readily absorbed in a social context: "Friends, neighbors, community participation provide high continuity of self definition despite retirement" (p. 281). Successful aging does not depend on activity (or disengagement) as such but on maintaining social networks, pursuits, and life-styles over time.

Narratologically considered, continuity theory offers virtually unlimited contingency: patterns of aging can vary from one personal identity to another. Such plasticity is undoubtedly an advantage in spinning individually tailored stories of aging, but from the standpoint of gerontology has the overwhelming disadvantage of dissolving its master categories—aging and the aged—into nothing but individuals: "The major difficulty with this theory is its solipsistic basis—there are potentially as many paths to happiness in later life as there are old people" (Estes, 1978:44). Gerontologists might enter this plot as advisory crafters and protectors of individualized patterns of aging, but to the extent that the reality of aging as a general process and the aged as the collective actant of that process is decomposed, gerontology itself is undermined and cannot be a coherent narrative presence in the world thus narrated. Continuity theory represents, therefore, an antigerontology narrative of aging and can function only as a resistance movement within the field as a whole. Certainly the field cannot articulate itself in its subject matter if aging is dispersed into anecdotal particularity and the aged reduced to nothing but different people with different personalities aging each in their own way (Novak, 1988:133). Without the aged as a narratably real collective actant there is not only little for gerontology to do in its communicative acts (its discourse), but little for it to be. This is a topic to which I will return in the next chapter. Meanwhile I will conclude the present discussion with a description of demography as the narrative center of the field of gerontology as a whole. The crux of narrative plots of the field and its master categories.

DEMOGRAPHY AS THE NARRATIVE CENTER
OF GERONTOLOGY

A human science, to be such, must create narratives about individual, typical, and collective actants. It must also, especially if it is a young science like gerontology, narrate its own coherence and its place in a larger scheme of things. I call this a field narrative, and its integrative thread a field plot.

Attention was drawn in the introduction to the strategic significance of demography in the field of gerontology as a whole, and, in Chapter 2, reference was made to the crucial role of demographic data in making aging and the aged possible and urgent objects of study, thus helping to found the field. The present discussion specifies the notion of strategic significance in terms of narrative centrality and shows in closer focus how demography provides a gathering place for the multiple, diverse topics of the field.

In gerontology's field narrative, the central subject around which events are circulated is not the aged but modern society. The events in question are threats, challenges, and pressures posed by the aged, the actant position to which it is assigned being that of an enemy to societal integration and orderliness. It is not a villain, to be sure, but an alarming presence nevertheless. Gerontology enters itself into the plot as mediator, adviser, reconciler, and helper between modern society and the aged, sometimes by name but more often as the narrative voice distributing predicates to actants, values to subjects and objects, and rationally conducting exchanges between them. In all this, demography supplies a narrative base from which to introduce other topics and show their pertinence as belonging to the same field.

Virtually every survey and introduction to gerontology opens it to view (i.e., to narrative account) by presenting national statistics on age groups. Description begins to turn to narrative when cutting points with an interpretable linguistic meaning are inserted into the figures. For example, Rathbone-McCuan and Havens (1988:9), opening a geron- tological comparison of the United States and Canada, say that the "arbi- trary cutting point" of age 65 is "meaningful in terms of the flow of benefits from public resources to groups in society." They proceed, in standard fashion, to define "population aging as a series of increases in the percentage of older persons in the total population" (p. 9). Popula- tion aging can now be used as a meaningful predicate of whole societies to help tell stories about them.

When the same interpretive value (the allocation of benefits from public resources) is applied at the other end of the age range, those under age 15 are equivalently significant to those 65 and over. The combined ratio of these two age groups to the group aged 15–64 is the age dependency ratio, supplying another demographic predicate with narratable meaning.

A story begins to emerge in showing that the age structure of a society is undergoing change. The two main changes are the aging of societies and the reshaping of age structures "from a wide-based, triangular pyra- mid to a more rectangular shape today" (Novak, 1988:60). These changes, formally specified in demographic transition theory, generate new problems and new events in modern societies, all having to do with dependency on others. Further predicates can now be added to give the narrative subject, modern society, a fuller character: predicates of bur- den, pressure, disorderliness, destabilization, and conflict. Cutler (1977), for example, speaks of the 18–64 age group as the "supporting" group and anticipates "substantial political conflict" as an expanding "older population" presses demands for medical care, transportation, housing, and economic well-being on the declining "supportive sectors of society" (p. 1013). Correlative with the demographic disorderliness of a rectangular age structure is the prospective economic disorderliness of an insufficient productive capacity to satisfy expectations, the financial disorderliness of insupportable tax burdens and insolvent pension funds, and the political disorderliness of intergenerational conflict.

Nor is this the end of the story. Gerontologists tell also of disorder in social life, in networks of care, and in the provision of specialized treat- ment for medical problems of old age. McKinney and de Vyver (1966:4) observe a "lack of established expectations and activities for the aged" and an "ambiguity of role patterns" leading to "a decrease in stability of social interaction and societal life generally as the number and proportion of aged in society increases." Treas (1981) argues that the decreased stability and size of family networks of interaction, associated with social mobility, geographical mobility, and declining fertility, have had "startling consequences" (p. 328) for care of the increasing numbers of relatives surviving into old and very old age: "kin networks can offer fewer options and resources when there are fewer members of the younger generations" (p. 329). Increasing longevity, registered in demographic data on mortality rates, is also disturbing for the provision of specialized health treatment. Wershow (1981) describes the problem of treating organic brain syndrome (OBS), an "irreversible disorder of learning and memory" (p. 176) associated with senility. It is reaching "epidemic" proportions in nursing homes and similar institutions: "the truly frightening dimensions of the problem of OBS are only beginning to emerge. The greatest proportional growth in the aged population is the rapid increase in *older* old people, i.e. those over 75 and 80 years of age" (p. 177).

Here then is a story of disorder: physical disorder, brain disorder, cognitive disorder, family disorder, social disorder, financial disorder, economic disorder, and political disorder—all narratably linked to demographic disorder. The entire narrative structure of gerontology is highly geared to demographic figures, such that even small turns of the latter generate large returns in interpretive commentary. In addition, demographic tabulation categories (under 15, 15–64, 55–64, 65–74, 75–84, 85+) can be transformed into analytic categories with theoretic significance (dependent populations, the supportive sector, the young–old, the old–old, for example), into legal, actuarial, and other institutional categories with policy significance, and into anthropomorphic actors with narrative significance. Demography thus underwrites, integrates, and provides a common currency of conceptual exchange for a discourse that is simultaneously scientific, applied, and humanly understandable. Narratologically and scientifically, demography is the strategic core of the field of gerontology.

One final point to make concerns the place of gerontology in its field narrative. Looking first at the narrative surface, the actant positions of protagonist and antagonist are filled by modern society and the aged, respectively (the order being reversed, however, when gerontology switches to advocacy of the aged). In this scenario, gerontology inscribes itself in the actant position of helpful intermediary:

> There has been a growing consciousness among demographers and planners alike that they need information on the elderly population to help plan for the needs of this group. (De Vos, 1987:32)

Gerontology is a multidisciplinary field that works to replace myth with fact, fear with knowledge, and confusion with understanding. (Novak, 1988:357)

The helpful intermediary role sketched here is illustrated in the argument developed by Messinger and Powell (1987) that "shrill expressions of alarm being expressed [in Canada] over . . . the economic burden of supporting the elderly" (p. 569) are uncalled for since the "GNP pie" will grow and the proportion of the pie needed to support the elderly may actually decrease. Nonetheless "as a safeguard" (p. 583) policy changes to encourage private sector pension plans and personal savings should be implemented. Clearly the helpful intermediary role has many different expressions and could be illustrated many times over in other materials. What is common to the role as such, however, is that it belongs to an actant position opened up by divergence and clash between the aged and society, which is to say, in narrative practice, between the predicates used to identify the other two actants. Without such predicates gerontology would have no intermediary role to play and the narrative articulation of the discipline would be thrown in question. Indeed it can be asked whether gerontology would be narratively possible without utterances of divergence and clash between the aged and modern society. This *is* the self-inscriptive narrative of the field.

The question of narrative possibility is sharpened if we shift attention from the surface plane of narration to the axis of communication running through it. All discourse makes something known and is, therefore, a communicative address by a subject possessing knowledge to a subject capable of receiving it: "The introduction and recognition of knowledge in the utterance are accomplished by the *actants of communication* (enunciator/enunciatee or emitter/receiver), even if they are very often mediated by the *actants of narration*" (Greimas and Courtés, 1989:568). Even though actants in the narrative plane may be endowed with partial knowledge, they do not know the whole picture. Only the knowledge of the enunciator is total and comprehensive, which is why "the fundamental axis of discourse is the one that goes from the enunciator to the enunciatee . . . the *knowledge-object* passes from one to the other, either directly and wholly, or through the mediation of actants present within the discourse (which can yield progressive acquisition, bit by bit, of knowledge by the enunciatee)" (Greimas and Courtés, 1989:569).

In *discipline* discourse, the enunciatee is an intended reader (a member of a presumed community of competences and interests), and the enunciator a voice of the discipline, an agent of a collective author, never just an individual writer. Gerontology voices itself, so I have argued, through utterances of divergence and clash between the aged and modern society. The implication is that gerontology, as presently constituted, cannot narratively occupy its subject matter without representing the aged as an antagonist–protagonist juxtaposed to modern society (or some part of it) as protagonist–antagonist. Of course, gerontology might be able to reconstitute itself on a different basis, but my inquiry is limited to What *is* gerontology? What else gerontology *might be* is another question, but it is one that can be properly approached only through interrogation of the present.

5

Dispersal and Integration of "The Aged" in Gerontological Discourse

I have argued that "aging" and "the aged" are the master categories of gerontology—they bound, organize, authorize, and collect topics into a single framework. Also, "the aged," due to its grammatical form (a substantive noun plus the definite article), is particularly important in giving referential security to the field as a whole. The term by its very structure projects something with objective standing, already there, and commonly seen. A matter of "recognition at sight" conveyed by "a knowing glance" (Hamilton, 1949:8, 13) between author and reader. Straightforward use and acceptance of the definite article plus "aged" confirms a prior acquaintance with a familiar entity. It is a linguistic structure of communication that indexes a taken-for-granted idealization of "coherence and determinateness" (Pollner, 1987:46). For example, Kreps (1966), discussing "employment policy and income maintenance for *the* aged," unproblematically indexes the object:

> Attempts to formulate policy dealing with *the* position of *the* aged must therefore . . . . (p. 137)
>
> progress has been slowed because of society's failure to agree on the goals of policy for *the* aged. (p. 137)
>
> The media for publicly transferring income to *the* aged are already established . . . . (p. 152, emphases added)

The concern of this chapter is with internal forces of the field making for disintegration of the master category, and with counteractive mechanisms of reintegration: a dialectic of dispersal and consolidation.

A phenomenal feature of gerontology is the sustenance of a unitary thought-object, the aged, in the face of dispersive pressures built into the linguistic field around it. Stated linguistically, this means preservation of the integrity of the definite article *the* in front of *aged* so that no serious referential doubt emerges about the existence of the denoted object. Questions may be raised and qualifications made but no radical doubt is sustained that somewhere in a presupposed social reality outside the category is the entity named by it. In other words, thoughts of the linguistically constituted nature of social reality may enter gerontological discussion but they will in the continuing event of discourse be suspended and erased. That doubts enter, either symptomatically or conceptually, is guaranteed by the reflexive relation of social reality to the linguistic medium. That they are limited, suspended, and erased is dictated by the ruling commitment of the discourse to referential stability and the other rationality requirements of substantive realism. The interplay of these two tendencies is as vital for the existence of gerontology as for any other social science; its presence in a text is indispensable for making that text reader redeemable *as* social science. It is a generic feature of that kind of writing.

SOURCES OF DISPERSIVE PRESSURE ON "*THE* AGED"

There are two sources of dispersive pressure internal to gerontology. (I do not deal here with external, contextual sources that are beyond the scope of the present study and belong to the contingencies rather than the inner constitution of gerontology.) Both sources derive from the general composition of a field of discipline discourse. It was proposed in Chapter 2 that any such field is built on two kinds of linguistic actions: (1) propositional statements articulating a subject matter, where the primary action is that of a translinguistic reference to something real made through a linguistic structure (prototypically a sentence), possessing sense, and (2) semiotic productions and circulations of meaning at the underlying level of the textual medium, where the unit of action is the sign and the primary action is signification through sign relations of difference, similarity, contrast, contiguity, opposition, and association.

Considered as nothing but a semiotic phenomenon, language is fraught with infinite openness and chronic lack of stability. Derrida (1978:280) says that signification is a process of "displacements and substitutions" but "the substitute does not substitute itself for anything which has somehow existed before it," consequently the "absence of the transcendental signified extends the domain and the play of signification infinitely." Eco (1976:68), recalling Charles Peirce's argument that the referent of a sign can only be another sign (a set, a category, a logical concept, etc.), draws attention to the infinite regression implied: "in order to establish what the interpretant of a sign is, it is necessary to name it by means of another sign which in turn has another interpretant to be named by another sign and so on. At this point there begins a process of *unlimited semiosis"* (original emphasis). The language user, semiotically conceived, is cast adrift in words and open to the opportunity (or threat) of infinite discursivity.

Semiosis is a fact of language—a fact played on by poets, punsters, psychoanalysts, and crossword riddlers, for example. It has also become, within the citadel of human science, a means of affrighting law-abiding inquirers going about their business. Free spirits, gathering under the banner, or perhaps one should say, playful neon light, of deconstruction and postmodernism, announce the end of discourse as we know it.[1] Such announcements are as true and as false as astronomy's view of the earth as a spinning rock hurtling through space. For those living on it, the earth is still as solid and dependable as ever. So also, language, for those who live in it and speak in sentences rather than merely signify in signs, is still massively dependable. The falsity of the scare, in both cases, lies in reducing a whole phenomenon to just one of its analytic facets. This is why Marx warned against the method of analytic abstraction from whole to parts and endorsed the reverse procedure of synthesizing whole thought-objects from abstracted elements: "The concrete is concrete because it is a combination of many determinations, i.e. a unity of diverse elements. In our thought it therefore appears as a process of synthesis . . . the abstract definitions lead to the reproduction of the concrete subject in the course of reasoning" (Marx, 1977:352). So, also, living language—language in use—must be thought as a configuration of semiotic, semantic, grammatical, rhetorical, and discursive elements, not reduced to just one of its components. With this proviso we can say that tendencies to dispersal (for example, metaphorical substitutions and metonymic displacements of a term) inhere in the semiotic substratum of a discourse, which is to say, where the discourse is written, in its textuality. This is the case with "the aged" in gerontology.

The second general source of dispersal of meaning in a field of discourse belongs to the discursive level itself. The wholeness of a field of discourse consists in bringing diverse particulars and manifold facts into a unitary scheme. Discursively this is done through the authority of master categories that project a comprehensible subject matter, this being a virtual pattern that diverse particulars can be taken to document. A master category operates at the textual level as an interpretant legisign toward which signification consistently and repeatedly turns to achieve accountable closure. "The aged" has this function in gerontology. The counterpart of integration, however, is articulation. Authority has to be

---

[1] Examples, and resistances, can be found in *Sociological Theory,* Fall 1990: Special Section on "Writing the Social Text."

extended and spread in order to be real; it needs to multiply its visible signs in order to be manifest. In discourse, a master category is compelled toward topical proliferation across the virtual extent of its domain, this being defined by all possible meanings (denotative and connotative, metaphorical and literal, descriptive and conceptual, applied and theoretical) of the category.

The immanent problem here is that of sustaining the referential identity of "*the* aged" in the course of such varied usages and through materials that have nothing self-evidently in common. In textual practice, the problem is that of controlling what language theorists call the *polysemy* of individual words and the *plurivocity* of whole discourses. Ricoeur (1976:17) observes that most words have more than one meaning and that a function of discourse is "to screen . . . the polysemy of our words and to reduce the plurality of possible interpretations . . . resulting from the unscreened polysemy of the words." However, discourse itself is liable to another form of uncertainty that confounds the screening process:

> A work of discourse is more than a linear sequence of sentences. It is a cumulative, holistic process. Since this specific structure of the work cannot be derived from that of the single sentences, the text as such has a kind of plurivocity, which is other than the polysemy of individual words, and other than the ambiguity of individual sentences. This textual plurivocity is typical of complex works of discourse and opens them to a plurality of considerations. (Ricoeur, 1976:76–77)

These general considerations have special pertinence for gerontology due to three features of the field previously observed: (1) the diversity of strands making up the foundations of the field, (2) the multidisciplinary character of the field, and (3) the dual commitment of gerontology to a scientific study of and participatory engagement in its subject matter, the latter being a constitutive interest of the field and not, therefore, amenable to common solutions like displacement to an applied branch attached to the main body of knowledge, or compartmentalization through a strong division between role of scientist and role of participant.

The combined problem of polysemic and plurivocal dispersal attending "*the* aged" is apparent in one of the standard textual overviews of the field: Binstock and Shanas' *Handbook of Aging and the Social Sciences* (2nd ed., 1985). A quick skimming of surface content reveals that "*the* aged" is all of the following: a social problem of family and nonfamily support (Chs. 4, 14, and 26), of housing (Ch. 15), and retirement rules and provisions (Ch. 15), a medical problem of treatment (Chs. 24, 25), an economic problem of support (Chs. 22, 23), a methodological problem of separating age effects from those of period and cohort (Ch. 11), a phase or period in a socially, culturally, biologically, and chronologically defined life course (Ch. 2), a structurally defined status and role situation (Chs. 3, 10, 12, 13), a cultural image of disease, decline, and death (Chs. 5, 6), a chronological classification in demographic analysis (Ch. 7), a social institution varying over historical time, especially modern time, and between cultures (Chs. 8, 9), a kind of minority group (Ch. 10), an income, ownership, and expenditure group (Ch. 16), a legal rights and entitlements category (Ch. 18), and a distinctive political actor (Ch. 19).

Now there is no reason to doubt the capacity of field practitioners to bring such diversity of reference into a single compass: the readable existence of the *Handbook* testifies to that. My point is that since there are continuous forces of dispersal operating on *"the* aged," subverting both its coherence and its referential security, there must also be a continuous work of repair, restoration, and reintegration going on—work that is simultaneously discursive and textual in nature, and that ensures the reality as well as the coherence of *"the* aged."

EXPRESSIONS OF THE DISPERSAL PROBLEM IN GERONTOLOGY

If it is true that a foundational category, "the aged," is under constant and strong dispersive pressure in the discursive operation of gerontology, this fact should be registered in expressions of difficulty and doubt by operatives of the field. This is certainly the case in the gerontology literature. A review of such expressions will help substantiate and extend the opening arguments of the chapter.

Gerontology consists to a large extent of processing policy materials from institutions of human care, public administration, and economic planning, and it is at this borderline we can first observe dispersive difficulties. It has become a standard observation in American gerontology, for example, that programs for the aged have become impossibly diverse:

> Our current agenda of public programs toward the aging is truly incredible for it includes virtually every aspect of human existence. (Binstock, 1981:154)

What becomes relevantly incredible for gerontology, however, is not just administrative overlap but the capacity of a single term, the aged, to conceptually embrace so many services and facilities as those now provided or to provide an adequate common denominator of them all.

Litwak (1980:87) gives the problem of administrative proliferation more of an epistemological cast in saying of community mental health centers providing treatment for the elderly that "the question arises as how best to ensure that the aged are included as a group." In other words, the question is how to sustain the categorical identity of being old above the individual treatment identity of being mentally ill. Should "services for the aged . . . be separated from the rest of the community mental health centers in a separate satellite structure" (Litwak, 1980:107), or should they be provided within existing centers as part of a "generalized mandate" (p. 107)? Are those under treatment to be rationally grasped as old people who are mentally ill, or as mentally ill people who happen to be old? The same questions arise with the aged who are poor, disabled, inadequately housed, and so on. Is an impoverished old person a rational knowledge-object primarily through being impoverished or through being old? Are the multifarious problems of old age really problems of being old, or only contingently and accidentally age related?

These uncertainties pass into academic gerontology. For example, Maddox and Campbell (1985) identify social integration and aging as a major topic of the field. The discussion is not, however, of a coherent scientific phenomenon but of widely assorted concerns from everyday knowledge, medical science, the caring professions, public administration, and the like. The evidence is "that older persons are more likely to be integrated than not. Chronological age per se is not an adequate predictor of social integration. . . . We see no necessary connection between age per se and actual or potential social integration on either theoretical or evidential grounds" (Maddox and Campbell, 1985:13). The same can be said of all other characteristics used to invest "the aged" with substantive meaning, raising doubt as to whether "there is any basis for asking questions specifically about the old at all" (Keith, 1985:238). In this context, it is relevant to recall, from the previous chapter, why American courts have refused to place age discrimination on the same legal footing as discrimination by race or national origin. Part of their argument has been that old age does not define "a discrete and insular group" (Eglit, 1985:533) because everyone goes through it. Moreover, there is no agreed age line at which old age begins, so the category has no definite boundary. Attempts to make age a criterion in jury selection have foundered on the fact that "with virtual unanimity the courts have rejected arguments that groups defined by age are cognizable" (Eglit, 1985:538). The legal judgment on the master category of gerontology is that it does not identify a substantive group, is a weak classification device, and is not cognizable: a potentially devastating dissolution of its cognitive authority. Interestingly enough, gerontologists often say similar things in their metamethodological reflections on the field, even though they must affirm the category in the actual conduct of their work. I take such contradictions between saying and doing to be symptoms of the countervailing pressures of dispersal and integration at work around "*the* aged" in gerontology.

Documenting the point further, there are frequent acknowledgments in the literature of the indefiniteness of the category. It is said to be contextually mutable and to be a relational rather than objective term. Mutability appears in the idea that "the aged" refers to a time bound, historically shaped cohort so that "the persons in the older age strata today are very different from older persons in the past and future" (Riley, 1985:371). It appears more strongly in social construction views of the aged:

> Despite its newness, we are apt to forget the novel meaning that became attached to the term *old age* in the twentieth century: a period in the life cycle prior to physiological decline, when productive activity ceases. This reconstruction of old age was made possible by the advent and expansion of the welfare state. The social, legal, and political constituency we now call 'the elderly' was created by social, political, and economic forces; and it can be destroyed or dramatically altered by those same forces. (Myles, 1986:213)

Acknowledgments of mutability confer a doubt amounting almost to irony in using the definite article in front of "elderly" or "aged." This is true also of acknowledgments that such terms have relational rather than objective meanings. Harvey Sacks (1989) draws attention to the distinction in comparing age and social class "category sets," on the one hand, with gender and race sets on the other. All of them are comprehensive sets that everyone has to belong to and that are used to monitor events and make conduct accountable (i.e., available to description, narration, and judgment). Whereas, however, gender and race categories have more or less the same application regardless of the category location of the user, this is not so with social class or age. If a 10 year old calls someone old, it has a different meaning than if a 60 year old says the same thing. The meaning is particular to the age relation of enunciator and object, not a standing feature of the object itself. Dependence of meaning on interactive context, like dependence on sociohistorical context, makes it difficult to speak with objective confidence of "the aged," and renders problematic the status of the designated object as a focus of scientific study.

The referential uncertainty about "the aged" induced by dissolution of the definiteness of the definite article is compounded in gerontology by admissions that the noun itself is only an arbitrary designation or a convenient marker and has no substantive meaning as such. The two

considerations are combined in Marshall (1987) who, in the manner
characteristic of gerontologists with a bent for critical reflection, hovers
between bracketing old age as just an arbitrary category of discourse and
accepting it as an intensely meaningful category of experience: "By extension of the idea that the personal experience of aging is conditioned
by the social context, it is critical to recognize that there are numerous
ways of growing up and growing old. Age itself is only a very crude
marker of one's life position" (p. 2).

Concessions of the conventionality and essential emptiness of the
signifier "the aged" abound in the literature. Maddox and Campbell
(1985:14) approvingly cite other opinions to the effect that "while chronological age can and does provide a convenient marker for locating
individuals in social space, the meaning of 'age' is in important ways a
dependent rather than an independent variable. The meaning of 'old'
varies by social and cultural context and is, at best, a relatively crude
marker of biological, psychological, and social capacity." They go on to
directly question "the utility of conceptualizing persons 65 years of age
and older as *the* elderly" (p. 17, original emphasis). Attempts have been
made to replace chronological with functional criteria of old age but
Streib (1985:351) calls this "a minority position" that he doubts will sup-
plant more convenient and, he says, "objective" chronological definitions. Age 65 is especially convenient because it corresponds both to a
demographic counting boundary and to institutional criteria for retirement and pensions. To the extent then that "the aged" is substantively
meaningful it is as an institutionally rather than scientifically formed
thought-object: "In American society we define old age chronologically . . . and place the onset of old age at 65. However, this age is
purely arbitrary. *It has no basis in reality* as the point at which a person
becomes old" (Harris, 1988:127, emphasis added).

We have then a master category, "the aged," which is admitted to be
unstable, crude, arbitrary, scientifically empty, and have no basis in
reality, yet which continues to function as an effective legisign in the
field of gerontological discourse all the same. We must now consider
some of the devices through which dispersal is controlled, dissolution
reversed, and substantive reality restored to the category.

DEVICES FOR GIVING COHERENCE AND REALITY
TO "THE AGED"

A distinction is to be made between devices whose primary function is
to stabilize usage of "the aged"—which I will call *integration devices,* and
those that serve primarily to endow the concept with real world

solidity—which I will call *objectification devices*. Obviously, there is functional overlap between the two types but there are good analytic reasons for treating them separately. Whereas integration devices concern the moves that can be made with a term, hence its *intra*linguistic *sense*, objectification devices concern projections of external correspondents to a term, hence its *extra*linguistic *reference*. (See Hendricks, 1976:174, on the contrast between "language-internal" sense and "language-external" reference in semantics.)

INTEGRATION DEVICES

Two devices of this kind are *synonymy* and *regulated subdivision*.

If polysemy is the runaway multiplication of different meanings around the same term, then synonymy, where the same meaning is conveyed through closely substitutable terms, can be regarded as a counteraction to polysemy (Ricoeur, 1977:114). In gerontology, the major synonym for "the aged" is "the elderly." Also common are "elderly people," "elderly population," "the old," and "older people." It is my impression that in modern gerontology "the elderly" and "elderly people" (or persons) are more often used than "the aged." However, the latter category owes its legisign authority to the fact that it nominalizes "aging," the ultimate collection category of the field, not to frequency of direct appearances. Sovereigns in discursive as much as in political domains govern more often through representatives than directly. Synonymy then spreads and extends a unitary legisign authority, the authority of "aging-and-the-aged" to rule the field, and does not divide or disperse it.

Having said this, however, it should also be acknowledged that "the elderly" and "elderly people" have distinctive semantic associations compared to "the aged," so that synonymy is more than identical repetition, it is a joining of semantic fields. Language theorists talk of the immediate field around a word as a sememe: "As we know, any word corresponds to a sememe, a set of distinctive semantic features, the semes, whose relationships determine that word's meaning (for example, the semes *human* and *female* are components of the sememe *woman*)" (Riffaterre, 1990:927). The point I wish to stress is that synonyms of "the aged" organize other sememes around the category, making it a more flexible linguistic joint around which to articulate topics on aging.

In advancing evidence for the point, it is helpful to recall an argument by Durgnat (1982) that semantic pathways around words develop through social usage and not simply through semiotic processes. Key words in ways of life are social institutions as well as units of sign

systems. Thus the English agricultural horse has acquired semantic concomitants such as plough, harness, field, and farmer, making it a different linguistic and social beast than the English riding horse (gentry,
hounds, fox hunting, jodhpurs). Likewise, "the elderly" has distinctive
concomitants compared to "the aged," allowing it to be used in a distinctive voice and tone even though the designatum is basically the same.

Illustration is provided by Fischer (1978). His project of comparing
reverential with phobic views of old age requires that the same thing be
described through completely opposite predicates. In general, Fischer
attaches neutral or negative predicates to "the old" or "the aged," and
positive predicates to "the elderly" or "elderly people." For example, he
speaks of "abhorrence of the aged" (p. 117), "trial and trouble for the
aged" (p. 153), and "poverty among the old" (p. 162), but "deference and
respect for elders" (p. 29), and "veneration for elderly people" (p. 32).
Sometimes the pattern is broken, for example, Fischer says "veneration
of the aged" (p. 37), so this is not a systematically planned division of
semantic labor. However, Fischer himself draws attention to the cultural
institution of "eldership" in various societies (pp. 8, 9, 13, 17, 38–41),
based on the equation of elder and better, and he criticizes Thoreau's
contempt for old age in terms of a contrast between synonyms:

> Here was a total reversal of traditional attitudes—a complete and decisive
> rejection of the ideal of 'veneration' and the institutions of 'eldership'. For
> Thoreau, 'the old', as he called them, were experienced only in the ways of
> failure, finished only in their forms of corruption. (Fischer, 1978:116)

I would note also of Fischer that he uses "elderly people" whenever he
wants to arouse the intersubjective understanding of the reader, for
example, "the plight of elderly people" (p. 156), and that he consistently
refers to "the elderly" when depicting the age group as a political actor
(pp. 176–177, 185–186, for example). This suggests that these two terms
are especially suited for humanistic and critical inflections of the gerontological voice. Those adopting the political economy approach (to be
examined in the next chapter), for example, speak on behalf of "the
elderly," "elderly people," and "older people" rather than "the aged."
Phillipson (1982) and Walker (1983) are cases in point.

Illustrations could be multiplied of how synonyms for "the aged" are
used in gerontology but a systematic study would require a separate
research project. For the present purpose I want only to be able to claim
that such synonyms allow for greater flexibility of tone and address than
would otherwise be possible—in particular, the addition of critical, humanist, and activist modes of address to objective and object-like accounts of "the aged."

The other integration device to be discussed is *regulated subdivision*. By this I mean the orderly break down of "the aged" into subgroups. The device responds to a particular problem in articulating the subject matter of the field: how to retain the integrity of legisign while admitting lack of unity in its referent. It is a measured defence, at the nominal level of measurement, against the thought that there may be no entity, no coherent thing corresponding to "*the* aged." The defense consists of naming subdivisions of the category and taking the whole category set to represent a heterogeneous entity. For this to work, however, the naming process must meet certain conditions of legible rationality. First, gerontological writing depends irreplaceably on demographics to ensure the legible rationality of aging and the aged. Consequently, the subdivisions must be referable to age categories. Second, however, age categories are not enough since it is precisely the suspicion of arbitrariness surrounding them which throws the rational coherence of "the aged" into doubt in the first place. They must, therefore, be supplemented with physical, behavioral, functional, or other substantive indicators of real difference. *Regulated* subdivision of "the aged" means *substantively rational* subdivision. Theorists of natural science often use a butchering metaphor to describe rational division. They contrast arbitrary conceptual distinctions with the "accommodation of language to the causal structure of the world . . . so that our linguistic categories 'cut the world at its joints'" (Boyd, 1979:358). Of course, this begs the larger question behind the present study of what such accommodation might mean where "the world" and its joints are themselves also linguistic, but I wish only to show how the unquestioned presupposition of something waiting to be cut informs the act of regulated subdivision and thus supplies a seemingly external authorization for it. Straightforward language unfailingly repairs the holes in reality that language in its reflexive moments makes.

Myers (1985:176) provides a typical gloss on the questionable homogeneity of "the aged": "there is a growing recognition that the aged population is a heterogeneous category of the total population in terms of such categories as age (sic), sex, race and ethnic composition, marital status, socioeconomic status and so on. This diversity is often not emphasized sufficiently when the older population is merely considered as a single category of the population consisting of persons 65 years of age and over." One way to emphasize the diversity of the older population would be to speak only of older people as individuals. This would, however, bring gerontology to a halt, since its discourse consists of articulating connections between individual and collective aging.

The discursive necessity of maintaining age categories is well illustrated by Grob (1986). Having drawn attention to the "arbitrary" nature of age classifications and wondered if indeed "it may very well be inap-

propriate to speak of the 'aged' " (p. 32), he proceeds to save the category
through rational subdivision:

> Note that I am addressing two different categories: the first is the elderly;
> the second is the varieties of individuals found within specific age groups.
> For to study 'the aged' is far too simplistic; we must understand how sex,
> class, race, and ethnicity—to cite only the most obvious—influence the
> condition of *the aged*. (Grob, 1986:33, emphasis added)

What I would stress here is the removal of doubt marks from "the
aged" following the introduction of cross-cutting categories whose substantive reality is so "obvious" as to go without saying. Conceivably
these categories too could be doubted for their arbitrariness but this
would not be fatal to the integrity of "the aged," since there is another
method of subdivision through which to preserve it. This applies behavioral and functional criteria of old age to the category. For example:

> Across the great range of differences among older people, it is useful for
> the policy maker to draw a distinction based on social competence and to
> distinguish the two groups who can be called, for convenience, the com-
> petent and the frail. It is important that this distinction is based, not on
> age, but on health and social characteristics. (Neugarten, 1987:393)

Notice how the opening concession to individual diversity is quickly
closed off by two proxies for the aged (the seemingly dispersed master
category): *the* competent and *the* frail. Neugarten instructs us not to hear
these as age categories, but since the entire context of discussion concerns being and becoming old, and since also the two groups are correlative with a chronologically marked distinction between the young–old
and old(est)–old that Neugarten (1974) herself pioneered, the instruction cannot be taken literally. "The aged" is still sovereign of the discourse, albeit in other words.

In conclusion, I would stress again the crucial role of noun forms in
stabilizing discourse. This is why "aging" alone cannot serve as the
master category and legisign of gerontology, but must be supplemented
by "the aged" (and its stand-ins). Goodrich (1987) has made the same
point regarding a language formation that, even more than gerontology,
is constrained to achieve stabilization: legal discourse. Goodrich ad-
dresses the very important question of how legal language generates an
authority to be accepted from within its own resources. The question,
that is, of the *intra*discursive production of authoritative words.
His answer specifies three features of legal language, the second of
which—its syntax of generalization—is directly relevant to the present
discussion.

Legal syntax is strikingly different from ordinary language in the extent to which it reverses the usual subject–verb–object order of direct declarative sentences, fills the left side theme position with impersonal terms, and deletes active subjects with specific identities acting in concrete circumstances in favor of categorical types embedded in generic processes and conditions. Basic to the syntax (which has also been attributed to science writing: Crystal and Davey, 1969; Gopnik, 1972; Gusfield, 1976) is a passive, nonagentive construction called nominalization: "A process, or verbal action, is expressed by a noun rather than a verb and assumes the identity of the participants in the process or action" (Goodrich, 1987:242, Fn. 62). As, for example, "the aged" replaces actual subjects of aging in sentences such as "The aged constitute a cohort that has passed through other ages," "The aged are discriminated against," or "The aged are not a homogeneous category." Nominalization need not place the named object in the lead-off position as in these examples, but such "thematization" of the noun-phrase reinforces the effects of distance, objectivity, and certainty conveyed by nominalization, as does the decontextualized and depersonalized form of depiction. Legal discourse, it is true, uses the syntax of generalization to endow words with a normative authority over concrete actions rather than, as in science, a cognitive authority over particular facts, but both are cases of strong discursive stabilization based on the same device. I do not say that nouns are exempt from underlying slippages of meaning at the semiotic level (all parts of speech are subject to semiosis), but at the level of discourse—where sentences rather than signs are the elementary unit of meaning—they do serve a significant stabilizing function through the syntax of generalization.

OBJECTIFICATION DEVICES

I wish to recall here the observation made in Chapter 4 that the subject matter of gerontology is articulated, in major degree, by metaphors of travel and passage. Such metaphors can be shown to play an important role in assuring the objective existence of "aging" and "the aged" for scientific study. They belong to a set of devices in gerontology through which reality effects are produced by the wordways of the field, so that what would otherwise be mere language is made into empirical discourse.

Beginning at the level of surface content, an important feature of travel and passage metaphors of growing old is that they allow time to be spatialized. Examples of spatialized time are timetables, appointment schedules, and clocks. All, as we have seen, are prominent concepts in gerontology. In the life course metaphor, aging is a chartable pathway in time, "a linking of successive roadmarkers as the traveler progresses" (Hagestad and Neugarten, 1985:45). The markers carry normative expectations of prescription, proscription, and permission such that the life course can be charted as "social timetables" of role and status transitions (Gee, 1987:266; Matthews, 1987:343), and as an appointed schedule of events marked on a "social clock" (Harris, 1988:165). Consequently, "one's position within the social timetables regarding life events" can be described as "off time/on time" (Harris, 1988:127). Analogous to the chartable pathway of the individual is "the cohort time trail . . . of living arrangement distributions laid down by a specific cohort" (Stone and Fletcher, 1987:288).

Events in *lived* time (Minkowski, 1970) pass away and cannot be collected together except in conceptual imagination. This is why Whorf (1956:139) calls *10 days* an "imaginary plural" in contrast to *10 men*, which is a "real plural" because the collection can be actually experienced in one group. According to Whorf, English grammar conflates real with imaginary plurals by applying the category of number equivalently to temporal events and spatial things, something not true, he argues, of Hopi grammar. In line with the principles of constitutive realism, I take this to mean that local linguistic devices exist for conferring the mark of spatial reality on representations of time—devices that might be specified to language communities like a field of study as well as to natural languages—and not that there is any absolute distinction between real and imaginary categories. Lucy (1985:84) understands him in much the same way: "Whorf called this 'objectification'—the treatment of intangibles such as time and cyclic sequences as if they were concrete, perceptible objects."

What needs to be added is that timetables, schedules, clocks, and other metaphorical representations of time *are* concrete, perceptible objects for someone using them, and so are time graphs and time-flow charts for someone reading a page of gerontology. There is no question here of creating illusions through smoke-and-mirror trickery, only of producing reality and knowledge effects through perceptible means of representation, means that are appropriate to some scene, circumstance, and realm of representation. Science is one such realm, and reading a science text one such circumstance and scene. Bordieu (1981:93–94) asserts that "science is possible only in a relation to time which is opposed to that of practice, it tends to ignore time and, in doing so, to reify practices." I accept most of this assertion, but it is misleading (and contradictory) to say that science has a relation to time that ignores it. Rather, the scientific representation of time, which is, we must recall, textually accomplished, transforms lived time into spatialized time and does so by negating constituent features of lived time. Whereas lived time is a sequential flux characterized by irreversible direction and immanent contingency, spatialized time in science is completely traversable and accommodates both synchronic pattern and causal necessity. Spatialized time in graphs and diagrams allows temporal process to be held in synoptic view, and thus made available for *review* and *research*— in other words, made an object of study.

Bordieu says that science has a time that is not only different from that of everyday life practice but opposed to it. If we take this to mean that scientifically represented time does not have an independent definition, but depends for its cognitive authority on negatively including lived time, then an important clue is offered to more general mechanisms of objectification in scientific discourse, therefore, in gerontology.

Time in science is a contrast structure of time standing against time passing. The standing–passing contrast structure has, however, a much wider application and deeper significance for discursive objectification than in the particular case of spatializing time. By seeing how else it is implemented, therefore, we can identify other objectification devices in discourse.

STANDING–PASSING STRUCTURES OF OBJECTIFICATION

When we perceive something standing constantly the same relative to adjacent change, we cannot help but see it as substantively real. This is a matter of direct cognitive apprehension rather than inferential reasoning. Deliberate reflection may of course call such a perception into question, but that is a secondary operation.

When Durkheim (1938:13) says that a social fact is to be recognized by its "external constraint," we can hear him to be making a grammatical statement (in Wittgenstein's sense) about the conditions under which a social fact is given to awareness, not just issuing a normative instruction to aspirant scientists. In this case, the production of a social fact in writing must reproduce those same conditions in literary form. My suggestion is that textual enactments of the standing–passing contrast structure are basic means of such reproduction. Durkheim's commitment to sociological positivism was too strong to allow him to pursue this kind of methodological reflection directly, even though his idea of sociology as a science using collective representations to study a reality composed of collective representations is an opening to do so. However, he does suggest two meanings of external constraint that can be given a textual interpretation.

One meaning of external constraint, in signifying a social fact, is that a way of thinking, feeling, or behaving exists "in its own right independent of its individual manifestations" (Durkheim, 1938:13). A social fact exists within yet beyond individual expressions of it, just as an average tendency is in yet beyond individual cases: "Currents of opinion . . . seem inseparable from the forms they take in individual cases. But statistics furnish us with the means of isolating them. They are, in fact, represented with considerable exactness by the rates of births, marriages, and suicides. . . . Since each of these figures contains all the individual cases indiscriminately, the individual circumstances which may have had a share in the production of the phenomenon are neutralized and, consequently, do not contribute to its determination" (Durkheim, 1938:8). In textual terms this criterion (or, I would say, producer) of facticity is any systematic juxtaposition, in the reading process, of superordinate general pattern to subordinate individual manifestations. This is accomplished in literary practices of summarizing the gist of evidence, diagramming causal pathways, juxtaposing a diagram with textual detail such as to make the diagram the inner pattern of the detail, instancing propositions, deriving typologies, and incorporating respondent quotations into interpretive commentaries. This kind of device is, I think, sufficiently familiar in general form not to require special illustration, and closer analysis would lead us into textual considerations too microscopic for our concern with the field features of gerontology as a whole.[2]

A second meaning of external constraint in Durkheim's account of social facticity is when a represented object, event, process, or state of affairs displays constancy amid changing views, impressions, and opinions of it. Durkheim contrasts the inconstancy of sense impressions, which he relates to preoccupation with concrete manifestations, with the constancy of objective perception:

> Indeed, the degree of objectivity of a sense perception is proportionate to the degree of stability of its object; for objectivity depends upon the existence of a constant and identical point of reference to which the representation can be referred and which permits the elimination of what is variable, and hence subjective, in it. (Durkheim, 1938:44)

Philosophically considered (i.e., in terms of a theory of method) this is an ontological pronouncement saying that the real is a constant referent which withstands changes of view and perspective. Textually considered, the regular, repeated circulation of the same denotative term

---

[2] For research data and further references to close, technical analyses of factual representation in scientific texts, see the special issue of *Human Studies*, April/July 1988.

through diverse semantic areas and applications will yield the effect of a constant, hence objective, point of reference.

In gerontology, representations of aging and the aged through seeking what is common in diverse beliefs, through criss-crossing between biological, psychological, sociological, and demographic aspects, or through presenting historical contrasts and cross- cultural differences, are not just conceptual operations of analysis and dissection, but textual affirmations of a standing reality. If it is possible to "look at . . . how aging differs in different societies . . . and how aging today differs from aging in the past" (Novak, 1988:28), then there is a presumptively real phenomenon of aging that transcends societal and historical variation— something that remains recognizably the same through here/there, now/then contrasts. By the same token, the unproblematic collection of multiple perspectives on aging and the aged into unitary handbooks, textbooks, and readers asserts the objective unity of what they are about. Maximization of variant perspective is indispensable to gerontology in ensuring the objectivity and coherence of its subject matter.

Even gerontologists who try to make social constructions of aging and the aged their primary concern do so by trading on the effect of objective existence that their own perspectivism evokes. Like labeling theorists in other areas of social research (especially crime and deviance), they accept enough of the idea of linguistic reality construction to formulate research problems—those having to do with stereotyping, societal perceptions, and the like—but, for the sake of securing a familiar methodological base built on the distinction between words and things, severely restrict the extent of its application. Achenbaum (1985), for example, advocates "humanistic research" on perceptions, images, and attitudes in the mass media, cultural artifacts, and ordinary language. But his aim is to "differentiate what is universal and unvarying about the meanings and experiences of growing old(er) from what is particular and time-bound" (Achenbaum, 1985:130). The rhetoric of method thus appeals to a taken-for-granted distinction between stable primary characteristics (the objects of discipline inquiry) and changeable secondary qualities (those immediately familiar to mundane reasoning). The distinction is expressed through conventional metaphors of shape and color: "humanistic gerontology emphasizes the extent to which modes of conceptualizing and expressing ideas perennially have shaped people's viewpoints of age. . . . Sometimes the terms we use to describe the aged are colored by our perceptions of the aging process. . . . Needless to say, ideas about age and aging are not shaped just by words. What people 'see' affects their perceptions" (Achenbaum, 1985:131).

Shape and color can be added to or subtracted from primary reality without fundamentally changing it because primary reality, by cultural consent, remains the same. Correspondingly, images of aging and the old may be shaped by words and colored by perceptions but underlying them are "the *same* physiological phenomena" (Achenbaum, 1985:131, emphasis added). This is why Achenbaum can ask seriously, though with unexplicated reservation: "To what extent have ideas, images, and stereotypes corresponded to the physical 'realities' of the human condition?" (pp. 130–131). The restriction of language to an additive function of labeling, shaping, and coloring extralinguistic things not only preserves the objectivist preconception of social reality from radical doubt but affirms it in reproducing the passing–standing structure of representation. Humanistic gerontology, like labeling theory, can study the effects of particular words and verbal formulas on what people think, feel, and do, but not address the full constitutive significance of language (including grammatical, syntactic and semiotic as well as semantic features) in the very composition of social reality.

THE STANDING–PASSING DEVICE IN AGE STRATIFICATION DISCOURSE

The age stratification approach in gerontology is especially rich in examples of the standing–passing structure of objectification and will serve to further document the device. I will draw on Riley (1985), a prominent exponent of the approach, for illustration (all page references following are to this source).

Riley makes a deliberate attempt to integrate two "previously disparate lines" (p. 370) of theory and research on age, thereby forming a coherent and solid object of discourse. The first line has focused on "the societal age structure" (p. 370), the second on "the dynamic aspects of social change, showing how each cohort of individuals has unique characteristics because of the particular historical events undergone" (p. 370). The standing–passing contrast is enacted here in the primary distinction between age structure and age process, and in the supplementary distinctions between cohorts undergoing historical events and individuals undergoing biographical and physiological events. Cohort is to historical event as standing is to passing, the individual is to biographical event as standing is to passing, and cohort is to the individual member as higher order (more constant, hence more objective) standing is to lower order (more variable, less objective) standing.

Riley's elaboration of the model proceeds through a series of distinctions indexing the same underlying formation of meaning: age-related roles are distinguished from persons of given ages, social change in age-related roles and role structures is distinguished from individual aging, "cohort flow" (p. 372) is distinguished from individual aging; and the overall social system is distinguished from "the age stratification system," which, in turn, "controls and continually changes the age structure of roles to which people are allocated" (p. 372).

That standing–passing is a grammatical formation rather than just a semantic distinction is proved by the fact that the same semantic unit can occupy either the standing or passing position, depending on what it is contrasted with, and that the semantic unit can refer either to a structure or a process. A structural concept can occupy the passing position as readily as a process concept can occupy the standing position. The positions are syntactic meaning spaces that confer significatory sense on the semantic units entering them over and above their referential sense. A cohort fills the standing position when used as a category to which individuals belong, but fills the passing position when used as an historical actant: "The life-course patterns of particular individuals are affected by the character of the cohort to which they belong and by those social, cultural, and environmental changes to which their cohort is exposed in moving through each of the successive age strata" (p. 374). Life-course patterns stand against individuals, cohorts stand against individuals, age strata stand against cohorts, and the entire propositional assembly stands to reason with the overwhelming obviousness of an object of perception. The syntactic formation grammatically duplicates sensory encounter, the very template of objective reality in our culture.

The ready adaptation of semantic units to the standing or passing position is important for the substantive coherence of discourse on aging and the aged. The same term can in a single statement turn from one position to the other, serving as a kind of pivot or relay through which to redouble the standing–passing formation in a continuous circuit. This is illustrated by the term *cohort* in the previous quotation. The following two quotations illustrate a variant of the device whereby a term is bivalently invested with standing-and-passing connotations rather than put to two uses successively. In the first extract, "collective movements" is the bivalent term, in the second, it is "the life course." Standing–passing positions carried by other terms are indicated in brackets:

Within a stratum [STANDING], people's similarity in age and cohort membership often signals mutuality of experiences, perceptions, and interests [PASSING] that may lead to integration or even to age-based groups and collective movements. (pp. 387–388)

In daily living [PASSING], small-group solidarity based on age, or 'age homophily' [STANDING] can be promoted where age peers are in a position to communicate about their similar tasks, needs, and problems and

about the exacerbation of these problems at stressful points in the life
course. (p. 388)

"Collective movements" and "the life course" are, in these contexts,
structures standing in relation to individual lives, but processes passing
in relation to structures outside aging. They provide places of discourse
(topoi) where the standing–passing positions can be joined as seam-
lessly as a perceived object to a direct act of perception. In discourse as
in perception, the constitutive innocence of the act ensures the externality of the object.

I will take one more example of the standing–passing objectification
device from Riley. Here we find bivalence thematized at the surface of
the text but metaphorically located in represented objects rather than
treated as a means of object production. Such displacement of productive resource into produced topic is, as ethnomethodologists have long
argued, a common way of protecting accounts from reflexive disturbance and thus maintaining their capacity to settle what is really going
on and really there for those concerned (Garfinkel, 1967:1–34; Wieder,
1974; Garfinkel et al., 1981; Pollner, 1987):

> The particular individuals composing any given age stratum are *not perma-*
> *nent residents in the stratum, but transients just passing through.* People *enter*
> the available roles and learn to perform them. But their role *occupancy* is
> limited. Soon they must *move on.* New cohorts take their place. . . . Many
> people *straddle* two *adjacent strata.* They are 'age incongruents'. (Riley,
> 1985:391, emphases added)

Temporary entry, role transiency, strata straddling, and age incongruents are said to derive from "the inevitability of the aging process
itself" (p. 391) and thus be *its* attributes, whereas they are, in textual
practice, elements of a rhetorical procedure for endowing the term *aging*
with evident and researchable objectivity in the reading process.

An additional observation to be drawn from the age stratification literature is that the capacity of the standing/passing device to objectify
aging is reinforced by its interpretive association with the macro–micro
distinction in social sciences, which is, in turn, metonymically close
to the traditional objective–subjective contrast in such fields. Riley
(1985:369), for example, says that age stratification theory sees "at the
macrolevel the age-stratified society (or smaller social institution) as
composed, at the microlevel, of individuals growing older in social roles
located at any given time in particular strata." Marshall (1987:2) extends
the contrast: "There is a 'micro' and a 'macro' side to aging, a personal
and a social side, an inside and an outside view." Subsequently, Mar-

shall associates the macro level with "social structure that provides the context for individual lives and social interaction" (p. 45). A chart of "micro," "linking," and "macro" theories of aging (p. 48) formalizes the contrast but at the same time its tabular format documents a continuous surface of discourse across which gerontology can move. Even personal aging inside individuals is thus incorporated into a publicly visible outside view along a continuum of researchable reality. Allowance for subjective aging thus projects the contrary existence of objective aging, voiced as contexts and structures, while the translation of the contrast into micro and macro levels of analysis binds both into a single, scientific vocabulary and yields a single object of study.

Lawton and Moss (1987), working with a double contrast between objective and interpersonal, as well as objective and subjective (though still within the macro–micro terms of discourse), take us back to the Durkheimian image of facticity used to initiate this entire discussion. Their interest is in informal networks of support, possibly "the most ubiquitous theme of gerontology today" (p. 92). They locate such networks at the micro level, thus allowing personal relations to be drawn by standard micro–macro formulas into the objectivating trajectory of scientific representation. An extra twist is added, however, by an ambivalent reintroduction of the objective–subjective distinction *within* the micro level: "For heuristic purposes, the objective environment consists of all that lies outside the skin of the person. One domain of the objective environment sector is the interpersonal environment, defined here as the aggregate of significant others who have some individual relationship . . . with the target person" (Lawton and Moss, 1987:93). They hesitate, however, to call informal networks purely objective because they involve intersubjective bonding: "Thus the ideal of the 'out there' aspect of the interpersonal environment is compromised by the intrapersonal factors involved in the selection of such a network" (p. 93). Thus, also, the linguistically constructed character of the "out there" aspect of interpersonal relations (and, I would say, of every "out there" aspect of all social reality) begins to appear. It is not that physical skin itself is a difference between objective and subjective social reality, but that the semantic marker "skin" is employed as a conventional linguistic signifier that *effects* the difference. Lawton and Moss virtually admit as much in their elaboration of what they call "a chink in the armor of any tight insistence that the interpersonal environment may be defined in purely objective terms" (p. 93).

The chink becomes evident in asking elderly people to name their networks. Naming (not skin boundary) objectifies the phenomenon for research purposes. Consequently, when naming is incomplete or vari-

able, the rendered phenomenon lacks full objective certainty. The in-
completeness is less in the case of family networks, where the "out-there
quality is perhaps more evident," than in "nonkin" networks, which are
therefore "more ambiguous" (p. 94). There are all sorts of people "with
whom we interact . . . but whom we simply do not think of when asked
to name our networks in any of the usual ways." The reference to *usual*
ways suggests the possibility of a solution to incomplete objectification:
the scientific invention of more complete ways to elicit naming. There is
"as yet no truly neutral question" that serves the purpose, but the prospect is left open. In this scientistically usual way, Lawton and Moss
reassert the ontological dogma that social facts exist out there in reality,
thus closing off reflection on the irremediable grounding of social facticity in language use that their own comments on questioning, naming,
and objective existence invite.

To sum up, the grammar of a social fact—conceived by Durkheim as
the criterion of external constraint—is implemented in gerontology
(though not of course exclusively here) in standard semantic demarca-
tions of standing–passing, outer–inner and macro–micro differences. It
is standard in the sense that any appropriate reader of gerontology—
that is, anyone possessing the membership competence, cultural and
specialized, to read into its texts what is presupposed, goes without
saying, and in no need of elaboration—will experience passage across
the standing–passing, outer–inner, or macro–micro differences as a social reality effect. I accept in this context an extreme view of what has
been called "the representation hypothesis" and so "deny the existence
of a macro-order apart from the macro-representations which are routinely accomplished in micro-social action" (Knorr-Cetina, 1981b:40–41).
Where fields of discourse are concerned, however, the microactions of
accomplishment are reading processes, and macroorders are accomplished in those actions through linguistic conjunctions of macro- and
microrepresentations. In analyzing the linguistic production of reality
and rationality effects, the communicative medium and setting need to
be taken into explicit account alongside semiotic, rhetorical, and discursive means of production. This is why I have emphasized the specifically
textual character of gerontology. Its production of reality and rationality
effects is tied to the literary medium and to a particular form of writing
lodged between human science, political advocacy, and humanistic interpretation. Gerontology writes aging and the aged into a definite and
highly authoritative form of legible existence. Like all social sciences it
studies a phenomenon that its own literary methods of appropriation
and representation make available for study. Gerontology is a specific
organization of such methods.

FRAMING AND OBJECTIFICATION

One further representation device, related to the standing–passing production of facticity, is the incorporation of mundane narratives of aging into discipline narratives. For example, eye-witness accounts of aging by elderly individuals, their relatives, friends, neighbors, and caretakers may be quoted verbatim within a coordinating framework of selective editing, reportage, interpretive commentary, and explanation. This yields a hierarchical nesting of more personal but less objective accounts within higher order accounts that are less real, in the personal sense, but more objective. The nesting structure as a whole thus confers reading effects of objective reality on any obviously relevant content presented through it—a content, that is, in conformity with the reading expectations of a genre, or the constitutive rules of a discourse.

Narrative framing is an objectification device found in all forms of writing based on veridicality: fictional or factual, scientific or nonscientific. The novels of Daniel Defoe, a pioneer of fictive realism, commonly begin with the author presenting himself in a preface as the editor of certain memoirs that happen to have come into his possession or that he has happened to have come across. The editor may offer explanations of gaps in the narrative—for example, the exhaustion of Robinson Crusoe's ink supply—thus reinforcing the sense of objective existence already conveyed by talk of contingent discovery. The act of novel creation is thus made into the constitutively innocent act of editing a first-hand report. As Goldknopf (1972:43) puts it: "Defoe has faked an editorial function to conceal an authorial one."

In talking of *factual* realism, I would say that the editorial function is performed rather than faked. It would be analytically wrong to say that journalistic reports, policy reports, and science reports are artistic fictions because this would miss their generic specificity. They produce reality effects to be taken seriously beyond the reading situation, whereas fictional simulations produce reality effects confined to the reading contract, and do so by playfully making their means of production a matter of admiration rather than incorporating them unreflexively into plain language representations of real world encounters. Fictive realism coquets with the literary production devices that in factual realism must not intrude, even after a reading has finished, since its cogency depends precisely on being an act of viewing, listening, seeing, repeating, and not, except trivially, one of reading.

The sociology of science has taken on new life since the 1970s by attending to the linguistic accomplishment of science in speech and writing (Latour and Woolgar, 1979, 1986; Knorr-Cetina, 1981b; Knorr-

Cetina and Mulkay, 1983; Lynch, 1985). The use of framing to achieve effects of objective reality has been noted by Knorr-Cetina (1981b) with regard both to narrating the authoritative writings of an area when presenting new findings, and to including the written traces of laboratory work in research reports. In both operations of the device, the effect of linguistic structure (the effect of framing per se) depends on the embedded content being appropriate. Cited writings need to be obviously authoritative so that their credibility is transferred in reading to the incorporative frame, and the report needs to be about *written* laboratory work: "The scientists who write a manuscript do not recall the research process and then proceed to summarize their recollections. Rather the link between the paper and the laboratory is provided by the written traces of laboratory work, which . . . form the source material around which the paper is constructed" (Knorr-Cetina, 1981b:130). Insertion of original spoken records of laboratory work in a research paper would break the conventional frame of a science report, opening it to a reflexive disruption of reality effects. This is exactly the procedure followed by the new sociologists of science to help turn scientific texts into analyzable accomplishments. The requirements of constitutive analysis are a reversal of the requirements of constitutive achievement.

In *social* science, the most obviously appropriate embedded content consists of participants' accounts of their experiences. The point was made in Chapter 4 that social science can only be done, and seen to be done, in appropriating mundane knowledge and ordinary language. The specific form taken by narrative framing in social science is then an implementation of this requirement. Respondent–informant–participant narratives evoke the knowledge of the reader as an ordinary member of society, while higher order narratives call out specialized knowledge. Textual incorporation of the former into the latter is simultaneously metanarrative and metaknowledge, which is to say, social science. As McHoul (1982:80) observes, trading on members' knowledge is no heresy to be condemned but "a crucial methodological resource."

Denzin (1990) helps describe how the resource is exploited in narrative framing by distinguishing between three levels of representation:

> When a subject describes her experiences in and through a second-order text, one furnished by the sociologist, *second-order empirical textual representation* occurs. When a subject's experiences, as given in a verbal account, are moved directly into a text without editing or interpretation, a *first-order empirical textual representation* is produced. When the sociologist rewrites the subject's experiences in his or her language and inserts representations of those experiences into a text, the result is another level of textual representation, called *analytic textuality*. (Denzin, 1990:212, original emphases)

Whereas, however, Denzin in his references to "a 'wild', uncontainable, worldly, flesh-and-blood version of the subject who continually eludes narrative capture" (1990:213) posits an elemental level of reality relative to which successive textual representations are increasingly distant and alien abstractions, I posit only local reality effects in distinct media, matrices, and contexts of production, without saying that some are more basic, true, or real than others. Embodied experience is a distinct zone and matrix of reality construction, not a privileged scene of reality relative to which textual representations are insubstantial replacements. Any concept of a reality beyond local hermeneutic productions of reality effects sets inquiry off on wild goose chases: a search for the sun outside a cave of shadows, for the ultimately real substructure of social superstructures, or for real things standing behind words.

To complete the discussion, I would note that objectification through framing is not confined to narratives, it is done also through direct references to levels of knowledge: a purely epistemological framing. Sacks (1989:257–258) observes something of the kind in introductory sociology textbooks where technical terms like "role" and "status" are slotted into basic sentences that students already understand as members of society without having done any sociology. Conversely, in professional discourse terms of membership knowledge are slotted into technical sentences, putting the frame device to scientific use in objectifying the ongoing account rather than to pedagogic use in substantializing technical terms. A conveniently compact example of epistemological framing is provided by Wister and Burch (1987). Reporting a study based on "personal interviews with 454 elderly persons (65 and over)" (p. 181), they construe the elderly persons (i.e., their interview protocols) as rational decision makers operating within a "decision frame" (p. 182), the frame being composed generally of "cultural knowledge and symbolism," and, more particularly, of "the decision-maker's conception of the acts, outcomes, and contingencies associated with a particular choice" (p. 182). With regard to the achievement of an objective contemplation of reality, the key is not the attribution of a decision frame to those interviewed but the inscription in the text of an epistemological viewing frame within which other's beliefs, conceptions, and so on are brought to view as a recessed vista of knowledge: like a landscape seen through an arch in mimetic painting. The actual terms of the inscription are various; in this particular text the phrase "it is argued here" serves the function:

> It is argued here that rationality in decision making can be thought of as a subjective process whereby individuals select and interpret information in a variety of ways . . .

It is argued here that social norms work through personal preferences in
affecting evaluations underlying decision outcomes. (Wister and Burch,
1987:182, 183)

"It is argued" marks the location of an enunciatory voice that is continuous with yet transcends what social members know, and what they can
show themselves to know in their voices. The "voice of the transcendental analyst" (Garfinkel et al., 1981:138) is for the corresponding reader a
linguistically composed interpretive posture, occupancy of which provides objective contemplation of the cultural knowledge and individual
rationality already lodged in the reader as a competent member of society. The rendered objectivity and reality of aging and the aged in gerontology writing, or of any social phenomenon in any field of social science, depend utterly on textual methods for turning prior membership
knowledge inside out, from interpretive resource to encountered topic.
A basic method is to syntactically and semantically frame such knowledge in the voice (which it itself a literary formation) of the transcendental analyst. This is the constitutive significance of conventional, formu-
laic passages such as *"Our data indicate that* elderly individuals view
'younger people' as frivolous in their spending habits" (Wister and
Burch, 1987:185). The framing effect is compounded when previous discipline knowledge of cultural and personal knowledge is introduced,
being then a frame within a frame: *"It has been stated that* the most
irrational aspect of the decision-making process is probably the limited
number of behavioral options that individuals perceive (Meeker, 1980).
This appears to be consistent with the previous discussion concerning the
propensity toward a routine or passive style of decision-making" (p.
186). In each of the three preceding passages, the emphasized phrases
(all emphases added) inscribe the voice of the transcendental analyst
(the scientific equivalent of the omniscient narrator in fiction), which
in turn gives voice to others (other researchers, elderly individuals).
The firmness of the hierarchical ordering and continuity of message endows the voice conducting the discourse with veridictory authority and
draws the reader into a tacit readiness to accept the truth value of what
is said. Greimas (1989e:653) calls such an agreement between the receiver and sender actants of a communication "the veridiction contract."
Maddox's further idea that veridiction be considered as "a type of
coherence" within a discourse, such that "the reservoir of knowledge
expands with the proliferation of voices" and increases the density
of the veridictory context (Maddox, 1989:664), receives direct endorsement in our account of the truth effects of narrative and epistemic
framing.

SUMMARY AND CONCLUSION

The chapter offers a further response to the question, What is gerontology? Gerontology is a discursive order built around the master categories aging and the aged, where the order emerges from a dialectic of dispersal and consolidation, unraveling and gathering, emptying and replenishing, deflation and reflation around the categories—in particular, around the definite article and substantive noun making up "the aged."

There are two major sources of dispersal: semiosis and extended application. The first stems from the linguistic underlay of the field and refers to semiotic displacements, deferments, and substitutions of meaning inherent to signification. The second belongs to the propositional level of the field and arises from the discursive imperative to establish the authority and relevance of its master categories (the legisigns of the field) throughout the domain they designate. The imperative dictates topical proliferation and a multiplication of applications around a category, opening it to variegated interpretations and immanent loss of referential cohesion. This process is especially marked in gerontology due to its diverse foundations, interdisciplinary character, and dual commitment to active intervention and scientific study.

The major consolidation devices, textually and discursively repairing the effects of semiosis and extended application, are of two kinds: integration devices and objectification devices. The former serve primarily to stabilize usage of a category and the latter to reflate a term threatened with emptiness (i.e., being reduced to the status of nothing but words); they do so by linguistically endowing the term with translinguistic reality effects. Two integration devices important in stabilizing the category of "the aged" in gerontology are synonymy and regulated subdivision. The verbal category "aging" is in turn lent both stability and substance through being nominalized in 'the aged' and its synonyms.

Objectification devices important for giving an effect of objective, translinguistic reality to the terms aging and the aged in gerontology include standing–passing structures of representation, and variants of these in perspectivism, narrative framing, and epistemic framing.

None of the restorative devices is in practice particularly startling or dramatic, nor can they be if they are to work. Their efficacy in stabilizing and substantializing a discourse in a course of reading depends, just like comparable devices identified in everyday speech by ethnomethodologists (e.g., Atkinson and Heritage, 1984), on being unremarkable and, in that sense, trivial. The reading effect of an objective discourse about external reality depends precisely on trivializing the reading act so that, using Hjelmslev's (1969) distinction, the plane of expression is invisibly absorbed into the plane of content.

In response to the irreverent but always relevant question, So what? that attends all social inquiry conducted within the realm of the already known (where all social inquiry begins and ends), I would give the same answer here as for the study as a whole. Gerontology makes old age a rationally accountable phenomenon through a definite structure of discourse. The organizing principles and constitutive processes of the structure operate as grammatical necessities and constraints on the representation of old age and, therefore, on recognizably rational knowledge, policy, and behavior concerning old age. Since it is the goal of gerontology to open up prospects and possibilities of rational orientation to old age by reflecting on limitations of knowledge, the reflective process should surely encompass internal limitations built into the organization and operation of gerontology itself. If, in our rational society, people called old are publicly treated according to the technical ways in which they are made known, and if those ways are set by certain rules of discourse and patterns of language, then it must surely be important, both ethically and practically, to identify them.

6

Openings and Closings to Critical Reflection in Gerontology

Specific openings to critical reflection are built into gerontology by its methodological commitment to scientific inquiry (meaning inquiry in the natural science mode). They include critical reflection on the factual accuracy of popular beliefs, the logical and empirical accuracy of theories, the interpretive adequacy of explanations, and the validity and reliability of measurements. The commonplaces of scientific method ensure places of prescribed critical reflection in the field. The very commitment, however, that allows and prescribes these openings carries with it presuppositions that act as serious closures on reflection.

First, there is the presupposition that social reality is something external to acts of knowing and doing, and can, therefore, be objectively represented in operational measures, intersubjectively comparable sense data, and law-like statements of causal structure. The burden of the argument in Chapter 2 was that the objectivist presupposition, referred to there as the substantialist image of reality, is contrary to a constructionist concept of reality and places severe limits on consideration of the latter. It might be allowed entry as a position to be argued with in metamethodological debate, or a reason for greater openness to qualitative data and actors' definitions, but it cannot in the normal conduct and normal textual practice of gerontology be seriously accepted. There the disciplinary organization and legible cogency of the field demand constant recourse to devices for objectifying and substantializing its subject matter, aging and the aged, such as those discussed in the previous chapter.

A second closure on critical reflection arises from the presupposition of the unity of science. More exactly, the axiomatic belief that below the evident differences between natural and social science there is a basic commonality justifying the transfer of methods from the former to the latter. A frequently used term for this belief is scientism. I prefer not to use it, however, since the term carries connotations of mechanically aping natural science, which obliterate in polemical caricature the self-same question aborted by the axiom that is being attacked, namely, What is the methodological difference between natural and social science?

To take the question seriously and open the pathway to reflection closed by faith in the unity of science, we must take to the limit the possible truth of the claim. Doing so demands a viable formulation of common ground between the subject matters of natural and social science, such that a methodological continuity reasonably follows. From the previous argument, this cannot be done by asserting that both subject matters are characterized by substantive, thing-like existence. This route leads only back to the closures of objectivism. It has, in any case, been undermined by contemporary studies of the history and sociology of natural science showing that neither the creation nor the acceptance and rejection of theories there can be explained by the idea of achieving correspondence to objectively given, external realities (Kuhn, 1970, 1977; Holton, 1978; Knorr et al., 1980; Knorr-Cetina and Mulkay, 1983). Even natural science proceeds through applying logical and empirical techniques to interpretive models of the world, to a world revealed in what Heelan (1983) calls the readable technologies of a science, not to an extrainterpretive reality: "the 'text' which science 'reads' is an artifact of scientific culture caused to be 'written' by Nature on human instruments within the controlled context of a human environment" (Heelan, 1983:188).

It follows from acknowledgment of the hermeneutic character of natural science inquiry that no strong distinction from social science can be made in terms of objectively existent versus interpretively constructed subject matters; both rest on the latter. The axiom of scientific unity, carrying with it the implication of a leader–follower, advanced–underdeveloped, senior–junior relation between natural and social science, can, from this standpoint, be reasserted in constructionist terms at the metamethodological level and leave the tutelary relationship between them intact. Since it is precisely through this relationship that the axiom places closure on critical reflection, no automatic suspension of closure is obtained by switching from an objectivist to a constructionist concept of knowledge and reality. It does, however, open the possibility of suspension if the "reading" relation between means and materials of interpretation can be shown to be significantly different in the two forms of science.

A clue to such a demonstration is provided by Heelan's observation above that the observation devices of natural science *cause* nature to be written on human instruments, *turning it* into a text readable in and through human language. Two implications are contained here. First, the possibility of causing nature to be written and read, proved in the practical success of science, implies that nature has a semiotic structure (something long asserted in the metaphor of the divinely authored Book of Nature, employed by Augustine, Galileo, Spinoza, and Einstein, among many others). Second, the technical difficulty of "reading" natural "texts," together with the authentic sense of discovery that attends their interpretation, indicates an encounter between heterogeneous semiotic systems, human and extrahuman, the latter arising outside the former but recordable and transformable into them. In contrast, the semiotic materials of social science are homogeneous with the linguistic means used to record and interpret them. Consequently, whereas the interpretive problem of natural science is to develop within human language means of deciphering semiotic systems outside itself, a problem it has solved through mathematical language, the problem of social science is exactly the opposite: how to achieve, within human language, sufficient distance from phenomena formed of human language to obtain an analytic grasp of them—a grasp, that is, that will be interpretively true to their meaning, yet not succumb to mere repetition of the already understood and a consequent degeneration of analysis either into triviality or ironic mockery, both of which are common accusations made against social science. The "reading" problem in social science arises, therefore, from reflexive closeness rather than translatory distance between the linguistic means and semiotic materials of study.

From the standpoint of an axiomatic commitment to the unity of science (for example, Jasso, 1988), the closeness of social science to ordinary language is a scientific defect to be overcome by mathematicization. The question of the *specific* "reading" demands of *social* science materials is thus silenced by methodological fiat from another realm. The materials are to be treated as if not already understood and being, therefore, in need of semiotic transformation to discover their sense. Simulation of the interpretive condition of natural science is used to define the demands of social science, thus closing off further reflection. The effect of the commitment can be seen in the response of gerontologists to persistent deviations of the field from natural science coherence, and to its continuing closeness to societal priorities. Both are attributed to lack of theory, and lack of theory is attributed to the youth and immaturity of the field:

> Social gerontology has been criticized as being too concerned with practical issues and problems confronting the aged. Many gerontologists believe that social gerontology has grown at the expense of a more theoretical orientation. (Kart and Maynard, 1981:1)

> Theory is a very small part of the social gerontological literature. . . . Few people in the field will be offended if I describe social gerontology as being young and somewhat immature. (Johnson, 1976:148–149)

Axiomatic belief in the unity of science predefines gerontology's internal lack of conceptual authority over its materials as a lack of the kind of authority any science ought to have, looks to the kind of theory found in natural science as the secret for establishing conceptual authority, and presupposes a development toward the natural science model of maturity with the passage of disciplinary time. The combination of submission to extrinsic standards of judgment and the comforting faith that scientific maturity is a function of time closes off questions of what scientific maturity might properly mean in social, cultural, and human sciences, what their linguistic relation to their materials should be, and whether there is a *necessary* closeness between the conceptual practices of such sciences and the practices making up their subject matters. It is the virtue of traditions such as hermeneutics (Gadamer, 1975; Dilthey, 1976; Ricoeur, 1971, 1974, 1978, 1986) and critical theory (Habermas, 1971) to have kept such questions open. The principles of constitutive realism (see Chapter 2), drawn in part from these traditions, are intended to serve the same purpose. These principles do not say that a contrary switch to denying any unity of science and asserting a totally interpretive, constructionist view of social science guarantees methodological reflection, this can lead to dogmatic impositions and cul-de-sacs of its own. Most damaging, perhaps, is the counterdogma that there is no basis of social reality except in what we subjectively and intersubjectively make of it; consequently, "there are as many varieties of reality as might be experienced by people" (Prus, 1990:356), no standards by which to judge one perception against the next, no possibility of analytic authority, no unifying theory, and no cumulative inquiry, only what Baldus (1990:470) criticizes as "radical sociological subjectivism." I agree with Baldus that unlimited relativism, taken to its extreme in postmodern, deconstructionist sociology, is parallel to objectivist, positivist sociology in leading to "intellectual closure" (p. 474) and another kind of "conceptual ritualism" (p. 473), with a resulting emasculation of the critical capacity of social science. But the principle that social reality is linguistically constructed dictates no such position, because human language is a union of collective system and individual performance, constraint and selection, object and subject, therefore a methodology based on the linguistic principle must contain the same contraries in unison. It is perfectly suited to the basic demand of critical reflection in social science, that of treading and retreading thin lines that are always in discursive practice being obliterated. In the following section, I will apply the principles of constitutive realism to the most sustained attempt at critical reflection in gerontology—the political ecnomomy approach—to show where and how it too imposes closures.

THE POLITICAL ECONOMY APPROACH IN GERONTOLOGY

The political economy approach has emerged at a border area between social gerontology and the neo-Marxian critical theory tradition in sociology. As such it has a specific mandate for critical reflection on the field, a mandate that combines an explanatory schema with an emancipatory project. The latter embraces not only elderly individuals caught up in the classificatory snares and institutional toils of social administration, but also gerontologists captured in the unexamined assumptions of their discourse.

The explanatory schema of the approach has three levels. It begins with causal determinants lodged in the economic structure of a society (more exactly, a nation-state), then moves through cultural categories of consciousness to individual level images, perceptions, and definitions. The first two levels are conceptually continuous with Marxian theory (which imparts a somewhat ironic twist to the restored name political economy, since Marxian theory originally developed as a *critique* of political economy); the third level borrows heavily from symbolic interaction theory in interpretive sociology.

Guillemard (1983:1) reports that a group of researchers attending a session of the Research Committee on Sociology of Aging, at the World Congress of Sociology, August 1978, in Uppsala, Sweden, found themselves in common disagreement with much "academic gerontology," and began discussing the development of a "political economy of aging." Apart from its political aquiescence (or perhaps as a part of it), academic gerontology was found to be methodologically wanting: it examines legislative programs separately instead of seeing them as parts of a whole strategy of public policy, it uncritically accepts a pluralist concept of power close to the ideological self-consciousness whereby capitalist societies represent themselves as democratic societies, and it fails to consider "the relationship between the policy making process and the larger class structure or the nature of the state apparatus" (Guillemard, 1983:4).

These failings of standard gerontology and the recommendation of Marxian structural analysis to solve them are standard features of the political economy approach. Olson (1982:xi) criticizes "liberal remedies," popular among gerontologists, because they "treat only the symptoms rather than fundamental causes of specific problems." The causes are rooted in market and class structures—"American capitalist institutions" (p. xi)—that elude the conceptual grasp of theories saturated with the very same preconceptions through which those structures are naturalized, euphemized, and kept safe from coherent view:

I assume that most gerontologists, and other policy analysts studying the
aged, while adept at cataloguing and describing the multitude of urgent
issues facing the elderly, fail to identify the roots of social ailments and the
limits to reform imposed by existing political, social, and economic institutions. (Olson, 1982:2)

What must be done is to analyze the "basic logic . . . of monopoly
capitalism" (p. 223) and critically confront the requisites of capitalist
production rather than uncritically reproducing those requisites in ideo-
logically constricted science.

Along the same lines, Estes (1983) describes some "dominant perceptions of reality" (p. 171) in American society that localize and individual-
ize problems of aging: the ethic of individual responsibility, the negative
view of centralized government, and the individualistic view of social
problems. Such perceptions "obscure an understanding of aging as a
socially generated problem and status, diverting attention from the social and political institutions that, in effect, produce many of the problems confronting the elderly today. . . . The political economy approach
is distinguished from the dominant gerontological perspective by viewing the problem of aging as a structural one" (Estes, 1983:177).

It is another standard feature of this approach that aging *is* a problem,
that being and becoming old are typically negative experiences, and that
the problem of aging is a social one, arising from causes amenable to
political intervention. Structural explanation is thus tied to an activist
emancipatory intent. Olson (1982:27) attributes "pernicious effects on
the elderly" to "deep transformations" in the American economy such
as "de-skilling," the "proletarianization of the work force," and forced
retirement. These can be traced to the intentional actions of human
agents—corporate capitalists and government planners—seeking to
sustain profit levels, accumulation, and productivity; the causes are,
therefore, amenable to counteractional intervention by other human
agents. Not, however, the interventions of "free-market conservatives
and liberal accommodationists" (p. 217), because they leave the framework of intentional action, the "basic logic of monopoly capitalism" (p.
219) intact. Only a dismantling of that logic through radical reforms
oriented to "democratic socialism" (p. 228) can decisively free the elderly from the traps of poverty, poor housing, inadequate health care,
and welfare state client dependency into which they are now systemically led. In the same vein, Phillipson (1982) describes the struggles
against poverty and ill health imposed on elderly people by "a web of
economic relations" (p. 154) spun from "the logic of capitalism as a
productive and social system" (p. 3), and urges a combination of militant
political action and the implementation of "a socialist social policy for

the elderly" (p. 165) to turn old age from a problem to "a natural part of the life-cycle" (p. 166).

The emancipatory intent of political economy is clearly expressed in its means as well as aims of intervention. For example, Phillipson (1982) regards it as essential to foster critical awareness and militant action among the elderly themselves. He welcomes radical groups such as the Gray Panthers and the development of a public voice among older people through "writings, speeches and pamphlets, urging those in later life to initiate a process of liberation" (p. 125). The political economy of aging has the same organizational, tutelary, and articulatory roles to play in this sphere of action as other neo-Marxian studies perform elsewhere, the entire assembly working to converge in a coherent coalition and single voice of radical reform.

The final component defining the political economy approach is acceptance of the significance of symbols, images, definitions, and other representations of reality in actually constituting reality. Some of this comes from the Marxian understanding of how ideological categories inform and sustain modes of social production, and some from the sociological tradition of symbolic interactionism and labeling theory, which has been readily grafted onto the approach. Phillipson (1982), for example, observes that older people "appear trapped within models of aging which emphasize the deterioration and loss of function accompanying old age" (p. 121). When this observation is placed in the context of the title of Phillipson's study, "Capitalism and the *Construction* of Old Age" (emphasis added), common ground begins to appear between the political economy approach and the present study, making it all the more important to come to critical terms with it. I will introduce a little more textual evidence to emphasize the apparent closeness between us.

A major figure in making explicit connections between critical gerontology and symbolic interactionism is Carroll Estes. Estes and Edmonds (1981:75) claim that the interactionist focus on "members of society as active creators of social reality" is a promising entry to power analysis because "power resides in the ability to control the definition of the situation." Estes (1978) explicitly locates old people in a situation defined for them by others, including orthodox gerontologists:

> Conceptualizations of aging and of the political potential of old people are indeed 'socially created' by those with power to devise paradigms, channel research, and interpret data; they define the basic problems of old age and delimit the range of possible individual and societal responses to these. (Estes, 1978:43)

Elsewhere, Estes (1979:x) adopts "the social construction of reality framework . . . concerned with delineating the perceptions and interests that shape societal priorities and policies for the old," and combines it with the "political economy perspective" on the determinants of perceptions, interests, and priorities. The major problems faced by the elderly are "socially constructed as a result of our conceptions of aging and the aged" (p. 1). These conceptions "take on an objective quality because people act as if they point to concrete realities" (p. 14). In her contribution to the Guillemard collection on political economy, Estes (1983) adds that there is a master conception of aging and the aged "that emerges within, reflects and bolsters the economic and political structure of society" (p. 169). The linguistic cast of Estes' formulation is repeated by other contributors to the collection, confirming the apparent closeness of this perspective to my own position, that of constitutive realism. For example, Guillemard (1983:76) says, "the emergence of a new 'territory' of social policy cannot be analyzed independently from the new social category—the elderly—which that policy presupposes as existing, and which views aging citizens in society as constituting a coherent and autonomous entity requiring the creation of a specific mode of management." Subsequently, she spells out the new mode of old age management in terms of new linguistic categories, just as another contributor, Walker (1983:151), draws attention to seemingly "neutral terms such as 'helping' and 'care'" which hide the reality of social definitions of old age being imposed on elderly people against their interests.

Obviously, I must find much to agree with in the political economy approach, especially in its attention to the language of social reality construction. In the following section, however, I will identify important closures built into the approach, continuous with those built into the orthodox gerontology it criticizes, thus justifying what might seem pedantic hedging in referring above to an *apparent* closeness between us.

CLOSURES AND PRECONSTRUCTIONS IN THE POLITICAL ECONOMY APPROACH

I will argue that the political economy of aging, despite its conceptual affirmations of reality construction, relies in its own practice on objectifying aging and the aged, thus reproducing the same basic closure as the standard gerontology it criticizes. Further, that objectification is a necessary (i.e., constitutive) feature of the approach, not something accidental or incidental to it. In part, this is because the political economy of aging aspires to *be* gerontology, not just a critical commentary on it, thus becoming liable to the constitutive features of that field: in particular, the objectification of its legisigns. Additionally, however, the approach draws on another field of discourse, Marxian analysis, which has its own protocols of objectification for producing knowledge effects. I will discuss these in terms of the material = substructure, consciousness = superstructure accounting schema, and the narrative code of political economy analysis.

To begin, I will illustrate objectivist preconstructions in political economy analysis. Preconstructions are utterances in discourse serving "to designate what relates to a previous, external or at any rate independent construction in opposition to what is 'constructed' by the utterance" (Pecheux, 1982:64); they are "lateral reminders of something that is already known from elsewhere" (p. 73). Such is the function served for gerontology by demographically, biologically, medically, legally, politically, economically, and common sensically known old age. Such also is the function of an already known logic of capitalism for the political economy approach. Additionally, by refracting the preconstructions of standard gerontology through its own preconstruction of capitalism, political economy recreates them, even though in its own terms, thus becoming not only an approach *to* gerontology but an accommodated approach *within* it. The interest is not in the fact that political economy analysis depends on preconstructions—this is a universal fact of all discourse whatsoever—but in its emergent closeness to what it would usurp and the fact that it too comes to depend on objectivist preconstructions of aging and the aged.

Take, for example, Estes' (1979) effort to integrate a social construction of aging approach with political economy analysis. She begins (p. 1) by saying that the major problems "faced by the elderly" are "socially constructed as a result of our conceptions of aging and the aged." It is, however, the problems that are constructed, not the elderly or the aged; the latter exist as presupposed objects of and for conception. The linguistic construction (and reproduction) of these objects in discourse (their's *and* our's) is glossed from reflection by the idea of social conceptions being draped around existent objects. This can be seen also in the neo-Marxian claim that "the aged are often processed and treated as a commodity" (p. 2). Again a problematic social meaning is hung on an unproblematically objective entity: the aged. The same structure of signification is repeated in the observation that social researchers and other professionals involved in aging policy are "actively engaged in modifying and structuring social reality for the aged." There is no notion of the aged being an utterly constructed social object, nor of utterances about "the aged" being means of reality construction. In ideology analysis, as in symbolic interactionism, there is only the idea of secondary qualities being added to existent things. Even the introduction of W. I. Thomas's dictum that "the perception of something as real makes it real in its consequences" (p. 13) is taken no further than the idea of negative stereotyping and labeling theory: labels, however, are stuck on a real object, the aged. Estes' halfway house position between a conceptual commitment to reality construction and a discursive commitment to objectivism is nicely illustrated in the following passage:

> This book explores *the problems of the elderly* from the basic premise that reality is socially constructed and that these constructions take on an objective quality because people act as if they point to concrete realities. *This is not to assert that the elderly face no problems independent of those that are perceived as real.* There are, indeed, phenomena associated with chronological aging and structural conditions *that may be said to be objectively real, regardless of how they are perceived.* Social action is, however, indivisible from the socially constructed ideas that define and provide images *of* these phenomena. (Estes, 1979:14, emphases added)

I would note finally of Estes, and of this entire approach, that in all passages designed to promote activist sympathy and an emancipatory intent, objectivist preconstruction becomes dominant, indicating its rhetorical indispensibility for this form of discourse. For example, the Older Americans Act expresses "interest-group liberalism . . . wherein . . . agencies, enjoying official status, define, validate, and institutionalize *the problems of the aged.* In a most blatant and tragic form, *the needs of the aged* are replaced by the needs of the agencies formed to serve *the aged*" (Estes, 1979:74, emphases added). In her peroration, Estes concludes that interest-group pluralism and the private bargaining model of politics need to be abandoned so that "the broader public interest and *the authentic interests of the aged*" (p. 75) can be satisfied (emphasis added).

In case it should be thought that Estes is not fully representative of political economy analysis, or that one instance is not enough, I will cite two other examples: Phillipson and Guillemard. These cases will also demonstrate the schematic equations, material = substructure, consciousness = superstructure, which, below any explicit theoretical endorsement, govern the performative code of political economy, that is, its performance in textual practice.

Phillipson (1982) announces a constructionist intent in the title of his study, but the actual performance is couched in terms of substantive realism. A scene-setting chapter (Chapter 2) on the demographic, financial, and health contexts of aging in capitalist society makes unhesitating use of visual metaphor to render unproblematic the denotative reference of "the elderly" and "the aged": "In the twentieth century, then, the aged have become more visible." (p. 8) . . . "Individually, we see the elderly trapped within an inevitable deterioration of their physical and mental powers; socially, we view them as a burden" (p. 11). The analytically significant point is how "the elderly" are viewed—"this stereotype deserves some correction and modification" (p. 11)—not the problem of the elderly being an object for viewing, or the methods by which that possibility is rendered an unremarkable presupposition. Political economy analysis exploits as a taken-for-granted resource what constitutive analysis takes as a topic.

The methodological closeness of political economy analysis to standard gerontology in depending on a substantively conceived subject matter is shown further in Phillipson's chapters (3, 4 and 5) on retirement. Chapter 3 describes "large-scale changes" (p. 39) in the economic substructure, "the labour market" (p. 16), and correlative manpower and welfare policies, whereas Chapters 4 and 5 consider "individual experiences and perceptions about ageing and retirement" (p. 39), thus projecting an overlay of consciousness on a visually secured substructure. When Phillipson comes to acknowledge his closeness to standard studies of retirement experiences, it is not to initiate a methodological break with them, but only to criticize them for tending "to isolate reactions to retirement from broader aspects of the economy and society" (p. 54). He proceeds then to describe these broader aspects as "the capitalist mode of production" (p. 55), and specify the relationship of consciousness to it in terms of reflection and structural causality: "while capitalism has created the preconditions for retirement in advance of physiological decline, it turns this period into one of insecurity. . . . This feeling of insecurity reflects the division between work and life . . . the hallmark of industrial and monopoly capitalism" (p. 57). The objectification and causal reification of capitalism are as basic to political economy discourse as that of the social system is to structural-functionalism. Both are amenable to moderate introductions of reality construction as long as these can be attributed to empirical processes within substantively real structures.

Guillemard (1983) has already been cited for her linguistic reference to the elderly as a new social category, and the strength of her commitment to constructionist theorizing makes all the more telling its subversion in discursive practice. She says, in thoroughly constitutive fashion, that it was "the development of retirement schemes that made possible . . . representation and identification of old age" as a homogeneous entity and an "object of public action" (p. 78). These and other marks of radical constructionism become erased, however, in objectivist references to "the state" taking action on "the elderly" in response to pressures from "the ruling class" and reflecting the needs of the economic system of capitalism. Trade union agitation in France in the early 1970s led *"the state* to alleviate the marginality . . . of *the elderly"* (p. 83); "the *evolution of social and economic structures"* (p. 89) has made necessary a new mode of old age management, "one that would be capable . . . of

adapting mentality to the new social system that was coming into being" (p. 94);
new programs on old age bear "the stamp of the socioeconomic situation
of the period" (p. 91), a period in which "the dynamics of *state action
regarding the elderly* are more directly determined by *the ruling class*,"
which "reflects a loss of autonomy by *the state* with respect to *society as a
whole* and a greater fusion of the political and administrative systems
with the centers of economic power" (p. 88, all emphases have been
added).

Within the substructure–superstructure schema of political economy
analysis, linguistic means of constructing social reality have to be located
in the consciousness = superstructure equation and made part of the
cultural dimension of society as a whole. Their status can never be more
than colorations, shapings, distortions, guises, and disguises of a prior
reality that is, in the last instance, economic. The typical metaphors of
their relation to reality are those of being imprints, reflexes, and reflections: "the welfare state in capitalist societies reflects the contradictions
embedded in those societies" (Walker, 1983:146); "the dominant societal
conception of aging and the aged . . . emerges within, reflects and bolsters the economic and political structure of society" (Estes, 1983:169);
"the treatment of social problems during the 1970's mirrored the task of
the decade—to put the economy on its feet" (Estes, 1983:171). In the
closures of mirroristic imagery, the existence of the mirror and the mir-
roring process are objectivistically hidden from reflection. In attributing
constitutive power to collective actants (the state, the ruling class, the
capitalist mode of production), the political economy approach surrenders to substantive realism and reaches the limit of its critical capacity.

I have referred to the substructure–superstructure schema as one
source of objectivist closure in political economy analysis, but there is
another. This is its commitment to a certain narrative code requiring
objectified and reified collective actants. This is a topic anticipated in the
discussion of narrative in Chapter 4, and I will do no more than provide
textual detailing of its operation in political economy writing.

The narratives of political economy are based on a stock cast of actants
from Marxian analysis. The actants include the exploiter–villain (always
played by capitalism and its metonymic extensions), the accomplice (frequently played by the state), the dupe (a deceived accomplice, variously
played but prominently including standard gerontology), the victim (the
poor, sick, disadvantaged old), the hero (critical gerontology, the political economy approach itself, figures prominently here), and the trans-
figured victim (in Marxian analysis, the proletariat become a revolution-
ary class for itself; in political economy narratives of aging, the aged
become an organized, articulate group for itself). The narrative code of
political economy analysis consists of these actants plus appropriate

action linkages between them, together with a regular source of contingent events to propel the action forward. Here the source is the capitalist economy and the events consist of its imperatives, crises, and ups and downs. Every narrative code includes a distinctive source of contingent events—destiny, fortune, individual character, supernatural intervention—that of political economy is the economic substructure of society. In total, the code provides a communicative pattern underwriting the textual performance and recognizable legibility of political economy analysis—in short, its reproduceable identity.

Standard gerontology typically occupies the dupe position in political economy narration. It is not deliberately exploitive like capitalism, but gets tricked into aiding the villain by gullibility and a blind good intent to help the aged. Olson (1982) notes incapacities of perception in standard gerontology, which she attributes to a liberal accommodationist view of society, "the perspective most prominent among gerontologists" (p. 15), and to a scientistic ideology of quantitative research. Both are structures of seeing that systematically screen out the operation of the system. The former selectively sees problems of all kinds as individual rather than collective, both in making causal analyses and in devising remedies. It also presupposes the political efficacy of groups of individuals, such as elderly people and their advocates, in the interest group bargaining process that is, for this perspective, political reality. Standard gerontology is duped into accepting and endorsing the pluralist, democratic guise of capitalism because it cannot see the structural causes of age-related problems, those built into labor market stratification and the like, nor, therefore, that the problems of the aged "are inherent in the normal functioning of American capitalism" (p. 21). The inability to see real causes or, consequently, to ask fundamental questions is compounded by scientist ideology:

> In their relentless pursuit of data, social scientists generally *confine the focus* of their research to *narrow* issues and questions that are quantifiable, while *ignoring* urgent problems that are less easily measured. The current thrust of gerontological research . . . promotes the idea of specific remedies to cure specific problems faced by the elderly. This *reductionist* approach *ignores* political and economic causes of social problems, and their linkages to broader structural issues. (Olson, 1982:211, emphases added)

Gerontology is identically characterized in all political economy narratives of aging. Another example is Walker (1983). Gerontology is dominated by the life-cycle approach to becoming old, leading to an uncritical acceptance that the low social and economic status of the elderly is "an inevitable consequence of advanced age" (p. 143). This view unseeingly "obscures inequalities between the elderly and younger people" (p. 144)

and has "largely overlooked" the role of the state "in creating and en-
hancing dependency" (p. 144). The gerontological literature further aids
and abets capitalism and its accomplice, the state, by discussing elderly
people "as if they were a distinct social minority, in isolation from social
values and processes, particularly the process of production" (p. 149). In
these and other ways of its writing, standard gerontology "reflects and
bolsters the economic and political structure of society" (Estes 1983:169).
In uncritically reflecting the status quo and its legitimating guises, gerontology the dupe merely duplicates capitalism instead of analyzing its
structures and revealing its strategems.

   The same combination of oversight, blindness, and gullibility is attributed to other figures in the dupe position: welfare agencies, social
workers, care planners, and socialist governments blinkered by mixed
economy mythology. Phillipson (1982) describes the good intent, high
hope, and false promise of the care policies initiated by the British Labour party in the late 1940s. He cites a proclamation of the Ministry of
Health, in its annual report of 1948–1949, that workhouses would be
replaced by group homes where old people could live as guests in a
small hotel instead of inmates in an institution, and comments sardon-
ically: "Unfortunately, the state, in the role of 'hotel manager', was to
change its policies on numerous occasions in the following years. The
guests could be forgiven for feeling unwelcome visitors, as the management made numerous attempts to run its establishment in a more profitable form" (p. 78). The commodity form, in other words, which is the
genetic code of capitalism, asserted itself in practice and turned the
reforms into hopeful illusions: "Hopes that the National Health Service
would radically improve the treatment of the elderly were not ful-
filled. . . . Consultants who worked in upgraded Poor Law hospitals
acted no differently from their colleagues elsewhere" (p. 88). Similarly,
the optimism surrounding the National Insurance System, introduced
by the Labour government in 1946, that old people would now be saved
from poverty, turned out to be naive hopefulness. Subsequent alterna-
tions of Labour and Conservative governments have affected the rhetoric of policy toward the elderly, but the logic of that policy remained
governed by cost–benefit calculations and constant pressures for expenditure cuts within the fiscal crises and economic priorities of a capitalist
society. Phillipson also assigns social workers to a dupe position, though
more in terms of indoctrinated blindness than gullible optimism. Social
workers are taught and trained in such a way that they adopt the "passive role" (p. 110) of operating administrative rules and helping elderly
people accept their social fate. Social work textbooks on the elderly
barely mention the structurally engendered struggles of old people for a
decent existence, treating the problems of aging as "private experiences"
(p. 110). Another version of standard gerontology thus enters the scene:

"This perspective, I would argue, has led traditional social work theorising on the elderly into a blind alley" (p. 110). A blind alley of ignoring, overlooking, and obscuring truths that would be embarrassing for capitalism and for its sometime dupe, sometimes willing accomplice, the state.

Capitalism is, then, a wily villain employing numerous dupes to mask its features and carry out its strategems. It is also, however, endowed, in the political economy narrative, with the tremendous powers of a giant. Olson (1982), for example, says that the capitalist class, while numerically a small minority, "holds vast economic and political power" (p. 21), and that "the modern capitalist system . . . is distinguished by the vast concentration of wealth and power in a few corporate and financial monopolies" (p. 23).

Narratively tensed against this formidable foe and the whole daunting array of accomplices and dupes is a victim endowed with seemingly hopeless weakness: the aged—in particular, the poor, sick, dependent aged: the frail elderly, elderly single women, elderly single black women, the lower class elderly, and the institutionalized elderly. The greater the accumulation of disadvantages and deficits in the victim, the more dramatic the narrative and the greater the task of salvation. This is provided for by attributing a latent active, powerful identity to the presently passive, weak victim, and assigning critical theory the role of truth-seeing, truth-telling mediator through whom the virtual identity can become actual. Multiple weaknesses are thus turned into an accumulated strength as the struggles against ageism, sexism, racism, and class inequality are made into mutually reinforcing moments of a single triumphant cause. Critical theory sees through surface appearances of prosperity to hosts of structural problems; the political economy of aging sees that the "myriad social ills associated with aging . . . have their roots in the same forces that generated the general U.S. economic crisis" (Olson, 1983:214). It sees also that "the specific problems experienced by the aged" are linked to "larger societal crises," and that they will only be solved all in one "through a progressive transformation of the American political economy" (Olson, 1983:217); Phillipson (1982) says that social workers, enlightened by critical theory, can help realize the strong virtual identity of the victimized elderly through passing on the insights of political economy: "we need to de-condition older people about their own limitations. . . . Older people should be helped as much as possible to determine for themselves a more radical programme of activities and social support" (p. 113). These former dupes of capitalism will also promote the practical side of practical–critical activity by helping set up neighborhood groups of elderly people, getting such groups to identify collective solutions to their seemingly individual problems, form networks, seek alliances, and otherwise politicize themselves: "The type of pensioner organizations most likely to emerge will be built along class lines or around single-issue campaigns. Broad coalitions may, for example, be built around campaigns over the adequacy of health and education facilities in retirement" (Phillipson, 1982:151).

I do not wish to question the factual adequacy or performative feasibility of the political economy approach, only to point out that the approach is conducted through a narrative code and conceptual schema dictating objectification of the aged as a collective entity and of aging as a collective process, a dual objectification bringing the approach close to the gerontological discourse it would replace. The relation of the political economy approach to the field of gerontology is, therefore, strangely close—a relation of the kind analysed by Miller (1979) as that of critic to host. It may be that the field is approached as a host in the sense of an enemy, but in being relied on for materials to feed critique the field becomes host in the sense of provider of sustenance, and even in the sense of consecrated bread distributed in communion to a congregation. Pieces of the host discourse are distributed and absorbed in the critical guest. Miller (1979:220–221) points out that the host as both eater and eaten contains the duality of both host and guest, while guest has the bifold sense of being friendly presence and alien intruder. The words host and guest have, in fact, the same etymological root, *ghos-ti*, providing linguistic reinforcement for the argument that in discourse a critic–guest is immanently liable to turn into the host. To this it can be added that gerontology is particularly suited to be the perfect host.

The frequently noted scientific immaturity of gerontology refers, among other things, to an absence of internal rigor and subsequent openness of boundary relations to other disciplines, making for considerable hospitality to others. Fischer (1978:194) observes that probably, "gerontology will never be a theoretical discipline in its own right, but rather a consumer of theory from other sciences.". Gerontology feeds from other tables but is, in turn, dispersed among them: guest and host together. Comparably, the political economy of aging feeds on gerontology and, in ingesting its accommodating host, becomes part of what it feeds on. Guest and host are enclosed in each other.

CONCLUSION

I will speak, in conclusion, of what textual analysis (which I take to be discourse analysis within a semiolinguistic framework) can contribute to social science. Taking to heart the warning of Douglas (1989) that hubris is the besetting sin of modern (he does not talk of postmodern) social science, it is fitting to be modest in making claims. Textual analysis is only a method of interpretive commentary, retracing the possibility of what others have already done; but that too is all any social science can be, and if the sole effect of textual analysis was to recall this limit, it would be worthwhile.

With regard to any particular social science, however, something more specific can be achieved. Textual analysis can articulate questions of method underlying the composition of a field and thus take new bearings on questions already articulated in the field itself. Our analysis of gerontology allows bearings to be taken on the following questions in and around the field: How can the hold of myths and stereotypes of old age be broken? What can be done to resist the subjection of elderly people to the formally rational treatments of science, technology, and bureaucracy? How is gerontology to resist capture in myths and stereo-types of old age? and How is gerontology to prevent itself from being another instrument of formal rationality in the service of bureaucratic "reglementations"? (Weber, 1978:642 defines these as normative instruc-tions to state officials on their duties that, unlike "claim norms," do not establish any rights of individuals.)

I would repeat that the point of raising such questions is not to evoke definitive answers, which would be a relapse into precisely the prescrip-tive hubris of theoretical reason that it is the virtue of textual analysis to puncture, but to take bearings. The least that methodological reflection can achieve is ground-clearing, restatement, and sensitivity to language traps; the most is to help wear away self-evidences and commonplaces so that "certain phrases can no longer be spoken so lightly, certain acts no longer, or at least no longer so unhesitatingly, performed" (Foucault, 1991:83).

Questions of capture in myth and stereotype are restated in textual analysis as the problem of how to work scientifically with, but not totally within, the linguistic bounds of membership knowledge. The bounds must be worked with, for writing to read as *social* science, yet worked against to be social *science*. The working question is the how, the linguis-tic means, of performing this closely contrary relation.

The common means in gerontology is to institute a linguistic segrega-tion, whereby certain segments of ordinary language are declared to be myths, stereotypes, or ideologies of aging, beyond the pale of scientific truth. The term ageism has come to designate language that is morally as well as scientifically beyond the pale. There are, then, empirical, logical, and moral procedures of linguistic segregation at work in gerontological writing, through which ordinary language, together with the structures of mundane reasoning carried in it, is worked with and against. A major policy implication of this mode of discourse is that many of the problems of old age, those due to misperception and misbelief, can be eased by

language correction: interventions to peel away wrong labels, demythol-
ogize aging, and destigmatize the aged. Language reform is made an
instrument of social reform. The reformist position is expressed, for
example, in Achenbaum's (1985) observations that "ageism needlessly
magnifies fears about growing old" (p. 144), and "stereotypic, inconsis-
tent, and erroneous perceptions of aging" (p. 144) distort decisions on
retirement, benefits, care, institutionalization, and so on, pointing to the
need to promote more correct language uses: "We can manipulate ideas
and images of age to fit new conditions, but there are limits to our ability
to create perceptions that have no foundation in historical traditions or
current realities . . . we must be prepared to challenge prevailing veri-
ties and alter our perceptions to conform more accurately to changing
circumstances" (Achenbaum, 1985:145). Estes (1979) advances the
reformist position in response to her own question, "what can we say
about the requisite construction of a new reality about old age?" (p. 227).
Again, new perceptions are to be created alongside rational accommodation to the "objective conditions" of being and becoming old. This points
toward a three-tiered reform program, the most important level of
which would be "major shifts in perceptions and structural alignments,
altering both the objective condition of the aged and the social processes
by which policies are made and implemented" (p. 241). The result of an
across the board reform "in our values, in our attitudes, in our behavior,
and in our actions toward the elderly" will be "a comprehensive national
policy on aging that does not segregate the elderly, stigmatize them or
place them in a dependent and depersonalized status" (Estes, 1979:247).

Through textual analysis, I have already pointed out the reliance of
such formulations on objectification of the elderly as a reality beyond the
name, limiting the role of linguistic reform to altering perceptions and
attitudinal colorations of that object. I have also pointed out (in Chapter
3) that objectification of the elderly is accomplished in gerontology
through a grammar of usage based on dependency. Consequently,
whatever gerontological reformers might recommend in the way of not
placing the elderly in a dependent position, their own discourse will
linguistically do just that, because this is how gerontology makes the
elderly an observable, measurable, rationally recognizable, scientifically
discussable thought-object. In this, it builds on grammatical foundations
common to societal language-games outside itself, thus ensuring relevance and cogency but, by the same token, not being able to radically
alter the position of the elderly. Loeb and Borgatta (1980:195) say that
"future research in aging will be more of what we have been doing
because we do not know how to do much different.". I take this to be a
confession of grammatical necessity rather than methodological mod-
esty. The situation is not, however, cast in stone, only in language.

Gerontology might radically change itself, and the position of the elderly, if it was able to reflect on the methods of reality and knowledge production constituting its field of operation. The office of textual analysis is to provide such reflection.

Following the same line of analysis, the reformist program in gerontology can be shown to contain false images of language, thereby inhibiting its purpose. The attacks on ageist vocabulary and the proposals to alter perceptions through lexical means imply that words contain thoughts and meanings. This is a mistaken picture of language, analyzed by Reddy (1979) as the conduit metaphor. According to the metaphor, writers or speakers put thoughts or feelings into words; these are transferred to readers or listeners who extract the contents from the words. The idea of words having insides filled with content cannot stand up to common sense consideration, still less to linguistic research. Furthermore, the very notion of an individual word containing a meaning is discredited by semiotic demonstrations of the dependence of linguistic values on structures of equivalence and difference between signs, that is, on sign relations rather than contents. Even so, the conduit metaphor retains a stubborn hold on our language habits. Reddy argues that its major framework easily extends into a minor one that dispenses with the concrete image of word as container, leaving thoughts and feelings to be simply sent into an external "idea space" (as in thoughts being put on paper, concepts floating around for decades, or ideas spreading through society). The contents thus achieve a reified existence outside any particular acts of making and interpreting meaning. One effect of this is to allow rational thought (if the reification might be permitted) to adopt an Archimedean position of truth and reality outside local, situated contexts and contingencies of language use. This is a position from which language can be brought into conformity with truth and reality and, in reformist spirit, used as an instrument of change.

The image of language, at least the language of social life, as something that can be instrumentally seized and used is another false picture of language. Any claim to knowledge must be made in some situated course of language use, so to claim an external position from which to judge the truth of language can only be the dogmatic assertion of a position forgetful or in denial of its own linguistic foundation. The instrumental picture, however noble the intent to do good, surrenders language to the Humpty Dumpty concept of meaning, where the only question is, Who is to be master? However, everything revealed by language scholars about contextual interpretation, indexical meaning, and indefinitely extending chains of signification denies the possibility of mastering language use, for whatever purpose, reformatory or otherwise.

Recalling the fate of Humpty Dumpty, it is important to stress that every attempt to leap outside human language in order to grasp and control it ends by falling back into it, since language is the reflexive medium of the leap and all the more elusive of control the more deliberately it is attempted.

One of the social implications of the conduit metaphor of language spelled out by Reddy is that problems of meaning tend to be blamed on the stupidity or malice of those using the language system, not on our false images of language. If thoughts and other meanings exist in external "idea space" and have that kind of intersubjectively available reality—the unproblematically available reality of things—then failures of meaning must be our or their fault. Accounts of ageism, delivered either as accusations of prejudice or confessions of guilt, illustrate the point.

Another practically relevant implication of the conduit picture is that the low expenditure of effort thought to be needed for clear communication is laid on senders (speakers and writers) rather than receivers (listeners and readers): "The function of the reader or listener is trivialized" (Reddy, 1979:308). This means that the constitutive significance of the interpretive moment, precisely the moment attended to by textual analysis of reading events, is bypassed. An extreme, and highly consequential, case of this is bureaucratic communication.

Ideally, a bureaucratic communication requires no interpretation, its meaning is entirely contained in itself and needs only to be retrieved. The human strangeness and estranging inhumanness of such language lies in a correlate of trivializing the interpretive moment. If it is rendered virtually redundant then so are the normal requirements of interpretation: the embedding of words in contextual acts of intended meaning by someone, for a purpose, subject to reactive negotiations of meaning. Hummel (1987:Ch. 4) in a series of contrasts with the language of social life, comments on the one-directionality of bureaucratic language, its closure to dialogue, its foreclosure of possible meanings, its indifference to contextual bearings, its removal from justifiable purpose, its erasure of personal authorship, and its detachment from situated contingencies of use. It is a functional conveyance of information, instructions, and "frozen decisions" (Simon, 1971).

The familiar Weberian theme of bureaucratization and the deadening triumph of formal over substantive rationality can, then, be given a linguistic meaning directly relevant to textual analysis and its possible role in making social life more sociable. Reflection on emergent accomplishments of discourse in acts of language membership must dwell on the immanent creativity of language and thus be enrolled in the wider task of keeping the interpretive moment of language open against bureaucratic, scientistic, or other closures. Weber himself, in a typically oblique sideglance to a value-relevant topic, "Excursus on the 'Cultivated Man'" (Weber, 1978:1001), adverts to the task in contrasting the educational demands of the professional expert and career bureaucrat (the specialist sender of communications) with those of the cultured person (the person capable of interpreting meanings). Comparably, Reddy (1979) calls attention to the difference between the conduit metaphor of language, making it seem that whatever we want to know can be stored in words (or other information depositories), and a "toolmakers paradigm," where what we want to know is constructed and reconstructed between us:

> We have the mistaken, conduit-metaphor influenced view that the more signals we can create, and the more signals we can preserve, the more ideas we can 'transfer' and 'store'. We neglect the crucial human ability to reconstruct thought patterns on the basis of signals and this ability founders. After all, 'extraction' is a trivial process, which does not require teaching past the rudimentary level. We have therefore, in fact, less culture—or certainly no more culture—than other, less mechanically inclined, ages have had." (Reddy, 1979:310)

I do not know what the full demands of cultural education might be in our time (we cannot simply return to classical models), but it is clear that they must include vitalization of the interpretive moment in human language, with appropriate allowance for differences between particular spheres, expressions, and forms of language. The demands of the moment are different in reading a social science discourse than reading a novel, a play, a piece of architecture, or a delicate situation. To meet them, it is essential to cultivate the ability to read social science reflectively.

Warnings such as those of Hummel and Reddy about the formal rationalization of language are amplified in Habermas (1987) as the colonization of the lifeworld, based on ordinary language, by political and economic systems of functional rationality, based on language-like symbols. They can be heard again in Foucault's (1977, 1982) nightmare vision of modern society as an incarceral archipelago formed from knowledge–power–language blocks of action. Sprinker (1980:14), commenting on the "innumerable mechanisms of the social machine, the microphysics of power" composing the archipelago, specifically includes the welfare bureaucracy, social administrators, and social scientists in the same complex.

In gerontology, the warnings are echoed in misgivings about "the routinizing tendencies of a bureaucratic society" (Van Tassel and Stearns, 1986:xx), and the displacement of informal by formal provisions of care, all of which forces forward the question of what might be done to resist such tendencies.

The approach taken here makes language use the key to anything that might be done but rejects as self-defeating any proposal to engineer policy reform or plan political action through instrumental uses of language, as in using theories to design better (more rational, more efficient, more effective) systems of care, organizing power movements around critical analysis, or seeking to alter language in order to redirect perceptions and control actions. All such uses, despite differences of rationale and political philosophy, share the same false picture of human language as an instrument, a picture belonging also to bureaucratic rationality and providing common ground between them. All such uses, therefore, regardless of intent, confirm gerontology in the service of the manipulated improvement of society, an ideal of social science that Bellah (1983)—following a distinction made by Shils (1980)—places in conflict with that of collective self-understanding. The former ideal approaches language from the outside, subordinating it to courses of strategic action in the framework of rational means–ends calculation; the latter operates within social language, making inquiry an extension of communicative action oriented to mutual presuppositions of truth, appropriateness, and truthfulness embedded in everyday speech, which is to say, in the possibility of understanding presupposed in beginning and continuing speech acts. (These contrasts are made by Habermas, 1979a:117–119, 209, 1984:94–101, 286–308). Radical remakers of the social order as much as status quo redesigners follow the strategic action ideal and belong, therefore, among those Habermas (1974:43) calls "engineers of the correct order." It is only a question of who is to be master.

Manipulated improvements of society belong to system rationality: to scientific knowledge, professional expertise, bureaucratic administration, and economic organization. De Certeau (1984) describes such apparatuses as places of control from which strategies, the games of the powerful, are conducted. These are, of course, linguistic and discursive as much as physical places. From within them relations of thought, power and will (i.e., strategies) are directed toward exterior objects fashioned in and by those relations: clients, customers, competitors, environments, research objects, and so on). Gerontology is such a place and the aged one such an object. Its strategies are deployed in the field of study it occupies—which has been our focus of attention—and in boundary transactions with policy-makers, program administrators, and care professionals. Radical (critical) gerontology would rearrange the place and alter the strategies but leave the pattern of power relations intact. De Certeau, in fact, sees little hope that counterstrategies can significantly change the organization of system power. He does not, however, recommend fatalistic quiescence. Built into everyday life and ordinary speech are what de Certeau calls tactics of the weak. These are ruses of avoidance, tricks of deflection, evasions of objectification, slippages of intention, ambivalence, ambiguity, irony, and paradox—an achievement of degrees of freedom—often inadvertently—by displacement rather than resistance. In linguistic terms, it is an exploitation of the reflexive properties and semiotic openness of human language.

From de Certeau's extreme divisions between the literary and the oral, text and voice—as in calling apparatuses of strategic power "the scriptural economy" and making the oral a subversive underground that eludes scriptural domination—it might seem that strategies of power belong entirely to writing and tactics of elusion entirely to speech. I would place textual analysis and all reflexive interpretation, however, among the tactical arts of the weak. Some warrant for this is provided in de Certeau's treatment of reading as an activity exterior to writing—one that he characterizes in terms of wandering nomadically across fields belonging to others, poaching from their domains, taking from their shelves, and otherwise infiltrating preconstructed orders. We might think, then, of a text as that which reading makes of a scriptural artifact. In terms of our opening distinctions, a discourse is the scriptural side of a field of writing and a text the readerly side. Textual analysis traverses the scriptural side in order to arrive at the other.

In a passage previously cited, Myles (1986:213), writing from the radical, political economy position, raises the intriguing possibility that "the elderly" as a social entity might disappear: "The social, legal, and political constituency we now call 'the elderly' was created by social, political, and economic forces; and it can be destroyed or dramatically altered by those same forces." It may be that the category will dissolve, but it will be through emergent shifts in language-games and the discursive conditions for producing reality and knowledge effects, changes beyond the scope of power strategies and planned intervention. Emergent shifts in language are more like natural events, even though they arise in and through human actions. "The elderly" might become obsolete, fade into disuse, or be erased—as Shelley imagines prints on a sandy beach being half erased by a wave, near the end of his poetic fragment "The Triumph of Life." The title is directly pertinent to our theme. It recalls the Weberian fear that social life will be deadened by the triumph of formal rationality, a fear still reverberating in the Habermasian struggle between system and lifeworld, and in de Certeau's celebration of everyday life practice against strategic exercises of mastery and control from central places of power, knowledge, and language. Gerontology echoes the struggle in the concern of critical and humanist practitioners to rescue individual elderly people from the objectifying, scientizing, bureau-

cratizing hold of "the elderly." The concern is valid but cannot be met by
adopting counterstrategies of destruction and alteration, mastery and
control, on behalf of the elderly. More crucially, the application of such
strategies to the language of social life for the sake of gaining instrumental leverage on an externally conceived social reality (the forces of society
referred to by Myles) threatens the very resource on which social life
depends. Language, like our other life resources, lends itself to rational
mastery and control, and to the undoubted benefits arising therefrom;
but, if seized strongly from without instead of worked with, from within, is liable to a deadening depletion. It is in this context that questions
of discourse such as What is gerontology? need to be asked.

Bibliography

Achenbaum, W. Andrew. 1978. *Images of Old Age in America 1790 to the Present.* Ann Arbor, MI: Institute of Gerontology.

Achenbaum, W. Andrew. 1985. "Societal Perceptions of Aging and the Aged." in Robert H. Binstock and Ethel Shanas, eds. *Handbook of Aging and the Social Sciences*, 2nd ed., 129–48. New York: Van Nostrand Reinhold.

Althusser, Louis. 1969. *For Marx.* London: Allen Lane.

Althusser, Louis, and E. Balibar. 1970. *Reading Capital.* London: New Left Books.

Antonucci, Toni C. 1985. "Personal Characteristics, Social Support, and Social Behavior." in *Handbook of Aging and the Social Sciences*, 2nd ed., Robert H. Binstock and Ethel Shanas, eds. New York: Van Nostrand Reinhold.

Atchley, Robert. 1981. "Retirement and Leisure Participation: Continuity or Crisis?" In Cary S. Kart and Barbara B. Manard, eds., *Aging in America: Readings in Social Gerontology*, 2nd. ed., 277–85. Sherman Oaks, CA: Alfred Sherman.

Atkinson, J. M., and J. C. Heritage. 1984. *Structures of Social Action: Studies in Conversation Analysis.* Cambridge: Cambridge University Press.

Austin, J. L. 1962. *How to Do Things with Words.* Oxford: Clarendon Press.

Baars, Jan. 1991. "The Challenge of Critical Gerontology: The Problem of Social Constitution." *Journal of Aging Studies* Fall (5):219–243.

Back, Kurt W., and Hans W. Baade. 1966. "The Social Meaning of Death and the Law." In John C. McKinney and F. T. de Vyver, eds., *Aging and Social Policy*, 302–29. New York: Appleton-Century-Crofts.

Bakhtin, M., and P. Medvedev. 1985 [1928]. *Formal Method in Literary Scholarship.* Cambridge, MA: Harvard University Press.

Baldus, Bernd. 1990. "In Defense of Theory: A Reply to Cheal and Prus." *Canadian Journal of Sociology* (15) Fall:470–475.

Barron, Milton. 1953. "Minority Group Characteristics of the Aged in American Society." *Journal of Gerontology* (8):477–482.

Barthes, Roland. 1967. *Elements of Semiology.* New York: Hill and Wang.

Barthes, Roland. 1981. "Theory of the Text." In R. Young, ed. *Untying the Text: A Post-Structural Reader.* London: Routledge and Kegan Paul.

Bazerman, Charles, and James Paradis, eds. 1991. *Textual Dynamics of the Professions.* Madison: University of Wisconsin Press.

Bellah, Robert N. 1983. "Social Science as Practical Reason." In Daniel Callahan and Bruce Jennings, eds. *Ethics, the Social Sciences, and Policy Analysis*, 37–64. New York: Plenum.

Bengston, Vern L., N. Cutler, D. Mangen, and V. Marshall. 1985. "Generations, Cohorts, and Relations between Age Groups." In Robert H. Binstock and

Ethel Shanas, eds. *Handbook of Aging and the Social Sciences*, 304–38. New York: Van Nostrand Reinhold.

Benhabib, S. 1984. "Epistomologies of Postmodernism." *New German Critique* (33):103–26.

Berry, Adrian. 1990. "The Tyranny of the Old." *The Sunday Telegraph*, February 4:19.

Binstock, Robert H. 1981. "Federal Policy toward the Aged: Its Inadequacies and its Politics." In Harold J. Wershow, ed. *Controversial Issues in Gerontology*, 153–58. New York: Springer.

Binstock, Robert H. 1983. "The Aged as Scapegoat." *The Gerontologist* (23):136–143.

Binstock, Robert H., and Ethel Shanas, eds. 1985. *Handbook of Aging and the Social Sciences*, 2nd ed. New York: Von Nostrand Reinhold.

Bird, Elizabeth S., and R. W. Dardenne. 1988. "Myth, Chronicle and Story: Exploring the Narrative Qualities of News." In James W. Carey, ed. *Media, Myths and Narratives*, 67–86. Newbury Park, CA: Sage.

Black, Max. 1979. "More about Metaphor." In Andrew Ortony, ed. *Metaphor and Thought*, 19–43. Cambridge: Cambridge University Press.

Bond, John. 1976. "Dependency and the Elderly: Problems of Conceptualization and Measurement." In Joep M. Munnichs and Wim J. van den Heuvel, eds. *Dependency or Interdependency in Old Age*, 11–23. The Hague: Martinus Nijkoff.

Bordieu, Pierre. 1981. "Structures, Strategies, and the Habitus." In Charles C. Lemert, ed. *French Sociology: Rupture and Renewal Since 1968*, 86–96. New York: Columbia University Press.

Bordieu, Pierre. 1988. "Flaubert's Point of View." *Critical Inquiry*, Spring (14):539–562.

Borgatta, Edgar F., and Neil G. McCluskey, eds. 1980. *Aging and Society*. Beverly Hills: Sage.

Borgatta, Edgar F., and R. J. Montgomery, eds. 1987. *Critical Issues in Aging Policy*. Beverly Hills: Sage.

Boyd, Richard. 1979. "Metaphor and Theory Change: What is 'Metaphor' a Metaphor for?" In A. Ortony, ed. *Metaphor and Thought*, Cambridge: Cambridge University Press.

Brown, Gillian, and George Yule. 1983. *Discourse Analysis*. Cambridge: Cambridge University Press.

Brown, Richard H. 1977. *A Poetic for Sociology*. Cambridge: Cambridge University Press.

Brown, Richard H., ed. 1992. *Writing the Social Text: Poetics and Politics in Social Science Discourse*. New York: Aldine de Gruyter.

Burke, Kenneth. 1954. *Permanence and Change*. Indianapolis: Bobbs-Merrill.

Butler, Robert N. 1969. "Age-ism: Another Form of Bigotry." *The Gerontologist* (9):243–246.

Cantor, Marjorie H. 1980. "The Informal Support System: Its Relevance in the Lives of the Elderly." In Edgar F. Borgatta and Neil G. McCluskey, eds. *Aging and Society*, 131–44. Beverly Hills: Sage.

Cantor, Marjorie H., and Virginia Little. 1985. "Aging and Social Care." In Robert H. Binstock and Ethel Shamas, eds. *Handbook of Aging and the Social Sciences*, New York: Van Nostrand Reinhold.

Cape, Elizabeth. 1987. "Aging Women in Rural Settings." In Victor W. Marshall, ed. *Aging in Canada: Social Perspectives*, 2nd ed., 84–99. Toronto: Fitzhenry and Whiteside.

Cerami, Anthony, H. Vlassara, and M. Brownlee. 1987. "Glucose and Aging." *Scientific American*, May:90–96.

Certeau, Michel de. 1984. *The Practice of Everyday Life*. Berkeley: University of California.

Chambers Twentieth Century Dictionary. 1972. London: W. and R. Chambers.

Chappell, Neena L. and Harold L. Orbach. 1986. "Socialization in Old Age: A Meadian Perspective." In Victor W. Marshall, ed. *Later Life: The Social Psychology of Aging*, 75–106. Beverly Hills, CA: Sage.

Chomsky, Naom. 1957. *Syntactic Structures*. The Hague: Mouton.

Chomsky, Naom. 1972. *Studies on Semantics in Generative Grammar*. The Hague: Mouton.

Cicourel, Aaron. 1974. *Cognitive Sociology*. London: Penguin.

Clark, Margaret. 1972. "Cultural Values and Dependency in Later Life." In D. O. Cowgill, et. al., eds. *Aging and Modernization*, 263–74. New York: Appleton-Century-Crofts.

Clifford, James, and George Marcus, eds. 1986. *Writing Culture: The Poetics and Politics of Ethnography*. Berkeley: University of California Press.

Cohen, Jonathan L. 1979. "The Semantics of Metaphor." In A. Ortony, ed. *Metaphor and Thought*, 64–77. Cambridge: Cambridge University Press.

Cole, Thomas R. 1986. "'Putting off the Old': Middle Class Morality, Antebellum Protestantism, and the Origins of Ageism." In David van Tassel and Peter N. Stearns, eds. *Old Age in a Bureaucratic Society*, 49–65. New York: Greenwood.

Connidis, Ingrid. 1987. "Life in Older Age: The View from the Top." In Victor W. Marshall, ed. *Aging in Canada: Social Perspectives*, 451–72. Toronto: Fitzhenry and Whiteside.

Cooper, William E., and John R. Ross. 1975. "World Order." In Robin E. Grossman, et al., eds. *Functionalism*. Chicago: Chicago Linguistic Society.

Cormican, Elin. 1980. "Social Work and Aging: A Review of the Literature and How It Is Changing." *International Journal of Aging and Human Development* 251–267.

Coulter, Jeff. 1989. *Mind in Action*. Atlantic Highlands, NJ: Humanities Press.

Crystal, D., and D. Davey. 1969. *Investigations of English Style*. Bloomington: Indiana University Press.

Cumming, Elaine. 1981. "Further Thoughts on the Theory of Disengagement." In Cary S. Kart and Barbara B. Manard, eds. *Aging in America: Readings in Social Gerontology*, 39–57. Sherman Oaks, CA: Alfred Sherman.

Cumming, Elaine, Lois Dean, and Isabel McCaffrey. 1960. "Disengagement: A Tentative Theory of Aging." *Sociometry* (23):25–35.

Cumming, Elaine, and William Henry. 1961. *Growing Old*. New York: Basic Books.

Cutler, Neil. 1977. "Demographic, Social-Psychological, and Political Factors in the Politics of Aging: A Foundation for Research in 'Political Gerontology'." *American Political Science Review* (71):1011–1025.

Danto, Arthur C. 1965. *The Analytic Philosophy of History*. Cambridge: Cambridge University Press.

Danto, Arthur C. 1985. *Narration and Knowledge*. New York: Columbia University Press.

Davies, Karen. 1985. "Health Care Policies and the Aged: Observations from the United States." In Robert H. Binstock and Ethel Shanas, eds. *Handbook of Aging and the Social Sciences*, 727–44. New York: Van Nostrand Reinhold.

Davis, Kingsley, and P. van den Oever. 1981. "Age Relations and Public Policy in Advanced Industrial Nations." *Population and Development Review* (7):1–18.

Denzin, Norman K. 1990. "Harold and Agnes: A Feminist Narrative Undoing." *Sociological Theory*, Fall:198–216.

Derrida, Jacques. 1978. *Writing and Difference*. Trans. by A. Bass. Chicago: University of Chicago Press.

De Vos, Susan. 1987. "Demography: A Source of Knowledge for Gerontology." In, Edgar F. Borgatta and R. J. Montgomery eds., *Critical Issues in Aging Policy*, Beverly Hills: Sage.

Douglas, Jack D. 1989. *The Myth of the Welfare State*. New Brunswick, NJ: Transaction.

Dowd, James J. 1981. "Aging as Exchange: A Preface to Theory." In Cary S. Kart and B. Manard, eds. *Aging in America: Readings in Social Gerontology*, Sherman Oaks, CA: Alfred Sherman. 58–78.

Drabek, Jan. 1989. *The Golden Revolution: Canadian Retirement Styles for the 1990's*. Toronto: Macmillan.

Drake, J. T. 1958. *The Aged in American Society*. New York: Ronald Press.

Durgnat, Raymond. 1982. "The Quick Brown Fox Jumps over the Clumsy Tank." *Poetics Today* 3 (Spring):5–30.

Durkheim, Emile. 1915 [1912]. *The Elementary Forms of the Religious Life*. Trans. by J. Swain. London: George Allen and Unwin.

Durkheim, Emile. 1938 [1895]. *The Rules of Sociological Method*. Trans. by S. Solovay and J. Mueller; G. Catlin, ed. Chicago: University of Chicago Press.

Durkheim, Emile. 1983 [1955]. *Pragmatism and Sociology*. Trans. by J. Whitehouse; J. Allcock, ed. Cambridge: Cambridge University Press.

Eco, Umberto. 1976. *A Theory of Semiotics*. Bloomington: Indiana University Press.

Edmondson, Ricca. 1984. *Rhetoric in Sociology*. London: Macmillan.

Eglit, Howard. 1985. "Age and the Law." In Robert H. Binstock and Ethel Shanas, eds., *Handbook of Aging and the Social Sciences*, 528–53. New York: Van Nostrand Reinhold.

Ehrlich, V. 1965. *Russian Formalism*, 2nd. rev. ed. New York: Humanities Press.

Eisdorfer, Carl, and Donna Cohen. 1980. "The Issue of Biological and Psychological Deficits." In, Edgar F. Borgatta and N. McCluskey, eds., *Aging and Society*, 49–70. Beverly Hills: Sage.

Erikson, Kai T. 1976. *Everything in its Path: Destruction of a Community in the Buffalo Creek Flood*. New York: Simon and Schuster.

Estes, Carroll L. 1978. "Political Gerontology." *Society*, July/August:43–49.

Estes, Carroll L. 1979. *The Aging Enterprise*. San Francisco: Jossey-Bass.

Estes, Carroll L. 1983. "Austerity and Aging in the United States: 1980 and Beyond." In Anne-Marie Guillemard, ed. *Old Age and the Welfare State*, 169–186. Beverly Hills: Sage.

Estes, Carroll L., and B. Edmonds. 1981. "Symbolic Interaction and Social Policy Analysis." *Symbolic Interaction* 4(1):75–86.

Estes, Carroll L., J. Swan and L. Gerard. 1982. "Dominant and Competing Paradigms in Gerontology." *Aging and Society* (2):151–164.

Fain, Haskell. 1990. "Some Comments on Stern's 'Narrative versus Description in Historiography'." *New Literary History* (21) Spring:569–574.

Finch, Henry le Roy. 1977. *Wittgenstein—The Later Philosophy*. Atlantic Highlands, NJ: Humanities Press.

Fischer, David H. 1978. *Growing Old in America*. Oxford: Oxford University Press.

Fish, Stanley E. 1980. *Is There a Text in this Class?* Cambridge, MA: Harvard University Press.

Forbes, William F., J. Jackson, and A. Kraus, eds. 1987. *Institutionalization of the Elderly in Canada*. Toronto: Butterworths.

Foucault, Michel. 1970. *The Order of Things*. Trans. by A. Sheridan. London: Tavistock.

Foucault, Michel. 1972. *The Archeology of Knowledge*. Trans. by A. Sheridan. London: Tavistock.

Foucault, Michel. 1977. *Discipline and Punish*. Trans. by A. Sheridan. London: Allen Lane.

Foucault, Michel. 1978. *The History of Sexuality*, Vol. 1. Trans. by R. Hurley. New York: Random House.

Foucault, Michel. 1980. *Power/Knowledge*. Edited by C. Gordon. New York: Pantheon.

Foucault, Michel. 1982. "The Subject and Power." In Hubert Dreyfus and Paul Rabinow, *Michel Foucault: Beyond Structuralism and Hermeneutics*, 208–26. Chicago: University of Chicago Press.

Foucault, Michel. 1991. "Questions of Methods." In G. Burchell, C. Gordon and P. Miller, eds. *The Foucault Effect*, 73–86. Chicago: University of Chicago Press.

Fowler, Roger. 1981. *Literature as Social Discourse*. London: Batsford Academic and Educational.

Frege, Gottlob. 1970. "On Sense and Reference." Trans. by Max Black. In P. Geach and M. Black, eds. *Translations from the Philosophical Writings of Gottlob Frege*, 56–78. Oxford: Basil Blackwell.

Friday, Paul. 1981. "Sanctioning in Sweden: An Overview." In Harold J. Wershow, ed. *Controversial Issues in Gerontology*, op. cit., 130–31. New York: Springer.

Gadamer, Hans-Georg. 1975. *Truth and Method*. London: Sheed and Ward.

Gadow, Sally. 1983. "Frailty and Strength: The Dialectic in Aging." *The Gerontologist* (23):144–47.

Garfinkel, Harold. 1967. *Studies in Ethnomethodology*. New York: Prentice-Hall.

Garfinkel, Harold. 1988. "Evidence for Locally Produced, Naturally Accountable Phenomena of Order." *Sociological Theory* (6) Spring:103–109.

Garfinkel, Harold, M. Lynch, and E. Livingstone. 1981. "The Work of a Discovering Science Construed with Materials from the Optically Discovered Pulsar." *Philosophy of the Social Sciences* (11):131–158.

Gee, Ellen. 1987. "Historical Change in the Family Life Course of Canadian Men and Women." Pp. 265–287, in *Aging in Canada: Social Perspectives*, Victor W. Marshall, ed. Toronto: Fitzhenry and Whiteside.

Gelfand, Donald E., and J. K. Olsen. 1983. *The Aging Network*. New York: Springer.

Giddens, Anthony. 1976. *New Rules of Sociological Method: A Positive Critique of Interpretative Sociologies*. New York: Basic Books.

Giddens, Anthony. 1979. *Central Problems in Social Theory: Action, Structure and Contradiction in Social Analysis*. Berkeley: University of California Press.

Giddens, Anthony. 1981. *A Contemporary Critique of Historical Materialism*, Vol. 1. Berkeley: University of California Press.

Giddens, Anthony. 1984. *The Constitution of Society*. Berkeley: University of California Press.

Gilbert, G. Nigel, and M. Mulkay. 1984. *Opening Pandora's Box: A Sociological Analysis of Scientists' Discourse*. Cambridge: Cambridge University Press.

Goldknopf, David. 1972. *The Life of the Novel*. Chicago: University of Chicago Press.

Goodman, Nelson. 1978. *Ways of Worldmaking*. Hassocks, Sussex: Harvester Press.

Goodrich, Peter. 1987. *Legal Discourse*. New York: St. Martin's.

Goody, Jack. 1986. *The Logic of Writing and the Organization of Society*. Cambridge: Cambridge University Press.

Gopnik, Myrna. 1972. *Linguistic Structures in Scientific Texts*. The Hague: Mouton.

Gordon, Jacob U. 1981. "The Black Caucus and Gerontology in Higher Education." In F. J. Berghorn, D. Schafer and Associates, eds. *The Dynamics of Aging*, 229–38. Boulder, CO: Westview Press.

Green, Bryan S. 1983. *Knowing the Poor*. London: Routledge and Kegan Paul.

Greimas, A. J. 1983 [1966]. *Structural Semantics*. Trans. by D. McDowell, R. Schleifer, and A. Velie. Lincoln: University of Nebraska Press.

Greimas, A. J. 1987. *On Meaning: Selected Writings in Semiotic Theory*. Minneapolis: University of Minnesota Press.

Greimas, A. J. 1989. (a) "On Meaning," 539–550; (b) "On Narrativity," 551–562; (c) (with Joseph Courtés) "The Cognitive Dimension of Narrative Discourse," 563–579; (d) "Description and Narrativity: 'The Piece of String'," 615–626; (e) "The Veridiction Contract," 651–660. *New Literary History*, Spring: Special Issue on Greimassian Semiotics.

Greimas, A. J., and Joseph Courtés. 1989. "The Cognitive Dimension of Narrative Discourse." *New Literary History* Spring:563–79.

Grice, H. P. 1975. "Logic and Conversation." In, P. Cole and J. Morgan, eds. *Syntax and Semantics 3: Speech Acts*, 41–58. New York: Academic Press.

Grob, Gerald N. 1986. "Explaining Old Age History: The Need for Empiricism." In D. van Tassel and P. N. Stearns, eds. *Old Age in a Bureaucratic Society*, 30–45. New York: Greenwood.

Guillemard, Anne-Marie ed. 1983. *Old Age and the Welfare State*. Beverley Hills: Sage.

Gusfield, Joseph. 1976. "The Literary Rhetoric of Science: Comedy and Pathos in Drinking Driver Research." *American Sociological Review* (41) February: 16–33.

Gustafson, Elizabeth. 1981. "Dying: The Career of the Nursing Home Patient." In C. Kart and B. Manard, eds. *Aging in America*, 503–18. Sherman Oaks, CA: Alfred Sherman.

Haber, Carole. 1986. "Geriatrics: A Specialty in Search of Specialists." In D. van Tassel and P. Stearns, eds. *Old Age in a Bureaucratic Society*, 66–84. New York: Greenwood.

Habermas, Jurgen. 1971. *Knowledge and Human Interests*. Boston: Beacon.

Habermas, Jurgen. 1974. *Theory and Practice*. London: Heinemann.

Habermas, Jurgen. 1975. *Legitimation Crisis*. Boston: Beacon.

Habermas, Jurgen. 1979a. *Communication and the Evolution of Society*. Boston: Beacon.

Habermas, Jurgen. 1979b. "History and Evolution." *Telos*, Spring:5–44.

Habermas, Jurgen. 1984. *The Theory of Communicative Action*, Vol. 1. Boston: Beacon.

Habermas, Jurgen. 1987. *The Theory of Communicative Action*, Vol. 2. Boston: Beacon.

Hagestad, Gunhild O., and Bernice L. Neugarten. 1985. "Age and the Life Course." In Robert H. Binstock and Ethel Shanas, eds. *Handbook of Aging and the Social Sciences*, 2nd ed. New York: Von Nostrand Reinhold.

Hamilton, George R. 1949. *The Tell-Tale Article*. London: Heinemann.

Hareven, Tamara. 1986. "Life-Course Transitions and Kin Assistance in Old Age: A Cohort Comparison." In D. van Tassel and P. Stearns, eds. *Old Age in a Bureaucratic Society*, 110–125. New York: Greenwood.

Harris, Diana K. 1988. *Dictionary of Gerontology*. Westport, CN: Greenwood.

Havens, Betty. 1980. "Differentiation of Unmet Needs Using Analysis by Age/Sex Cohorts." In, Victor W. Marshall, ed., *Aging in Canada*, 208–234. Toronto: Fitzhenry and Whiteside.

Hawthorne, Nathaniel. 1987. *Selected Tales and Sketches*. New York: Penguin.

Hazan, Haim. 1988. "'Course' Versus 'Cycle': On the Understanding of Understanding Aging." *Journal of Aging Studies* (2):1–11.

Hazelrigg, Lawrence. 1989. *Social Science and the Challenge of Relativism*, 2 vols. Tallahassee: Florida State University Press.

Heath, Stephen. 1972. *The Nouveau Roman*. Philadelphia: Temple University Press.

Heelan, Patrick. 1983. "Natural Science as a Hermeneutic of Instrumentation." *Philosophy of Science*, June:181–204.

Hendricks, William O. 1976. *Grammars of Style and Styles of Grammar*. New York: North Holland.

Henry, Jules. 1966. "Personality and Aging—with Special Reference to Hospitals for the Aged Poor." In J. McKinney and F. de Vyver, eds. *Aging and Social Policy*, 281–301. New York: Appleton-Century-Crofts.

Hjelmslev, Louis. 1969. *Prolegomena to a Theory of Language*. Madison: University of Wisconsin Press.

Holton, Gerald, ed. 1978. *The Scientific Imagination: Case Studies*. Cambridge: Cambridge University Press.

Homans, George C. 1961. *Social Behavior: Its Elementary Forms*. New York: Harcourt, Brace and World.

Hudson, Robert B., and John Strate. 1985. "Aging and Political Systems." In, Robert H. Binstock and E. Shanas, eds., *Handbook of Aging and the Social Sciences*, 554–85. New York: Van Nostrand Reinhold.

Hughes, Charles C. 1985. "Introduction." In Ronald C. Simons and Charles C. Hughes, eds. *The Culture-Bound Syndromes*, 3–24. Boston: D. Reidel.

Hummel, Ralph. 1987. *The Bureaucratic Experience*, 3rd ed. New York: St. Martin's.

Hunter, Albert, ed. 1991. *The Rhetoric of Social Research*. New Brunswick, NJ: Rutgers University Press.

Jakobson, Roman. 1956. *Fundamentals of Language*. The Hague: Mouton.

Jakobson, Roman. 1960. "Closing Statement: Linguistics and Poetics." In T. Sebeok, ed. *Style in Language*. Cambridge, MA: MIT Press.

Jameson, Fredric. 1972. *The Prison-House of Language*. London: Routledge and Kegan Paul.

Jameson, Fredric. 1987. "Foreword." In A. J. Greimas, *On Meaning: Selected Writings in Semiotic Theory*, vi–xxii. Minneapolis: University of Minnesota Press.

Jasso, G. 1988. "Principles of Theoretical Analysis." *Sociological Theory* (6) Spring:1–20.

Johnson, Malcom. 1976. "That Was Your Life: A Biographical Approach to Later Life." In J. Munnichs and W. van den Heuvel, eds., *Dependency or Interdependency in Old Age*, 147–61. The Hague: Martinus Nijkoff.

Kalish, Richard A. 1966. "A Continuum of Subjectively Perceived Death." *The Gerontologist* (6):73–76.

Kalish, Richard A. 1981. "Toward a Philosophy of Mature Aging." In, H. J. Wershow, ed., *Controversial Issues in Gerontology*, 233–42. New York: Springer.

Kane, Robert L., and Rosalie A. Kane. 1981. "Alternatives to Institutional Care for the Elderly: Beyond the Dichotomy." In, C. S. Kart and B. Manard, eds., *Aging in America: Readings in Social Gerontology*, 472–92. Sherman Oaks: Alfred Sherman.

Kart, Cary S., and Barbara B. Manard, eds. 1981. *Aging in America: Readings in Social Gerontology*, 2nd ed. Sherman Oaks, CA: Alfred Sherman.

Karttunen, L., and S. Peters. 1979. "Conventional Implicature." In C.-K. Oh and D. A. Dineen, eds. *Syntax and Semantics Volume II: Presupposition*. New York: Academic Press.

Keith, Jennie. 1985. "Age in Anthropological Research." In Robert H. Binstock and Ethel Shanas, eds. *Handbook of Aging and the Social Sciences*, 231–63. New York: Van Nostrand.

Keith, William M., and Richard A. Cherwitz. 1989. "Objectivity, Disagreement, and the Rhetoric of Inquiry." In, Herbert W. Simons, ed., *Rhetoric in the Human Sciences*, 195–210. Newbury Park, CA: Sage.

Kieras, David, E. 1985. "Thematic Processes in the Comprehension of Technical Prose." In Bruce K. Britton and John B. Black, eds. *Understanding Expository Text*. Hillsdale, NJ: Lawrence Erlbaum.

Kitzinger, Celia. 1987. *The Social Construction of Lesbianism*. Newbury Park, CA: Sage.

Knorr, Karen, R. Krohn, and R. Whitley, eds. 1980. *The Social Process of Scientific Investigation*. Boston: Dordrecht.

Knorr-Cetina, Karen. 1981a. "Introduction." In K. Knorr-Cetina and A. Cicourel, eds., *Advances in Social Theory and Methodology: Toward an Integration of Micro- and Macro-Sociologies*. 1–50. London: Routledge and Kegan Paul.

Knorr-Cetina, Karen. 1981b. *The Manufacture of Knowledge*. Oxford: Pergamon.

Knorr-Cetina, Karen, and M. Mulkay, eds. 1983. *Science Observed: Perspectives in the Social Study of Science*. London: Sage.

Koestler, Arthur. 1964. *The Act of Creation*. New York: Macmillan.

Kreps, Juanito M. 1966. "Employment Policy and Income Maintenance for the Elderly." In J. McKinney and F. de Vyver, eds. *Aging and Social Policy*, 136–57. New York: Appleton-Century-Crofts.

Kubler-Ross, Elizabeth. 1969. *On Death and Dying*. New York: Macmillan.

Kuhn, Thomas S. 1970. *The Structure of Scientific Revolutions*, 2nd ed. Chicago: University of Chicago Press.

Kuhn, Thomas S. 1977. *The Essential Tension*. Chicago: University of Chicago Press.

Lakoff, George and Mark Johnson. 1980. *Metaphors We Live By*. Chicago: University of Chicago Press.

Langer, Suzanne. 1948. *Philosophy in a New Key*. New York: Mentor.

Laslett, Peter. 1985. "Societal Development and Aging." In R. H. Binstock and E. Shanas, eds., *Handbook of Aging and the Social Sciences*, 199–230. New York: Van Nostrand Reinhold.

Laslett, Peter. 1987. "The Emergence of the Third Age." *Aging and Society* (7):133–60.

Latour, B., and S. Woolgar. 1979. *Laboratory Life: The Social Construction of Scientific Facts*. Beverly Hills: Sage.

Latour, B., and S. Woolgar. 1986. *Laboratory Life: The Social Construction of Scientific Facts*, 2nd ed. Princeton: Princeton University Press.

Law, John, ed. 1986. *Power, Action and Belief. A New Sociology of Knowledge?* London: Routledge.

Lawton, M. Powell. 1985. "Housing and Living Environments of Older People." In R. H. Binstock and E. Shanas, eds. *Handbook of Aging and the Social Sciences*, 450–78. New York: Van Nostrand Reinhold.

Lawton, M. Powell and Miriam Moss. 1987. "The Social Relationships of Older People." In Edgar F. Borgatta and Rhonda J. V. Montgomery, eds. *Critical Issues in Aging Policy*, 91–126. Beverly Hills: Sage.

Lemon, Bruce W., Vern L. Bergston, and James A. Peterson. 1981. "An Exploration of the Activity Theory of Aging: Activity Types and Life Satisfaction among In-Movers to a Retirement Community." In, C. Kart and B. Manard, eds., *Aging in America*, op. cit., 15–38. Sherman Oaks, CA: Alfred Sherman.

Levin, Samuel R. 1979. "Standard Approaches to Metaphor and a Proposal for Literary Metaphor." In A. Ortony, ed. *Metaphor and Thought*, 124–35. Cambridge: Cambridge University Press.

Levinson, S. C. 1983. *Pragmatics*. Cambridge: Cambridge University Press.

Litwak, E. 1980. "Research Patterns in the Health of the Elderly: The Community

Mental Health Center." In E. Borgatta and N. McCluskey, eds. *Aging and Society*, 79–130. Beverly Hills: Sage.

Loeb, Martin B., and Edgar F. Borgatta. 1980. "Values and Future Needs for Research." In E. Borgatta and N. McCluskey, eds. *Aging and Society*, 195–212. Beverly Hills: Sage.

Luborsky, Martin R. 1990. "Alchemists' Visions: Cultural Norms in Eliciting and Analyzing Life History Narratives." *Journal of Aging Studies* (4):17–29.

Lucy, John A. 1985. "Whorf's View of the Linguistic Mediation of Thought." In Elizabeth Mertz and Richard J. Parmentier, eds. *Semiotic Mediation: Sociocultural and Psychological Perspectives*. 73–97. New York: Academic Press.

Lynch, M. 1985. *Art and Artifact in Laboratory Science*. London: Routledge and Kegan Paul.

Lyotard, J. F. 1984. *The Postmodern Condition*. Manchester: Manchester University Press.

McClosky, Donald N. 1985. *The Rhetoric of Economics*. Madison: University of Wisconsin.

McClosky, Donald N. 1990. *If You're So Smart: The Narrative of Economic Expertise*. Chicago: University of Chicago Press.

McDaniel, Susan. 1986. *Canada's Aging Population*. Toronto: Butterworths.

McHoul, A. W. 1982. *Telling How Texts Talk*. London: Routledge and Kegan Paul.

McKee, Patrick, 1982. *Philosophical Foundations of Gerontology*. New York: Human Sciences Press.

McKinney, John C., and Frank T. de Vyver, eds. 1966. *Aging and Social Policy*. New York: Appleton-Century-Crofts.

Maddox, Donald. 1989. "Veridiction, Verification, Verifications: Reflections on Methodology." *New Literary History* (20), Spring:661–678.

Maddox, George L., and Richard T. Campbell. 1985. "Scope, Concepts and Methods in the Study of Aging." In R. H. Binstock and E. Shanas, eds. *Handbook of Aging and the Social Sciences*, 3–31. New York: Van Nostrand Reinhold.

Manheimer, Ronald J. 1989. "The Narrative Quest in Qualitative Gerontology." *Journal of Aging Studies* (3):231–252.

Marano, M. 1985. "The Windigo Psychosis among Northern Algonkian Tribes." In Ronald C. Simons and Charles C. Hughes, eds. *The Culture-Bound Syndromes*, 411–48. Boston: D. Reidel.

Marshall, Victor W. ed. 1980. *Aging in Canada*. Toronto: Fitzhenry and Whiteside.

Marshall, Victor W. ed. 1986. *Later Life: The Social Psychology of Aging*. Beverley Hills, CA: Sage.

Marshall, Victor W. ed. 1987. *Aging in Canada: Social Perspectives*, 2nd ed. Toronto: Fitzhenry and Whiteside.

Marx, Karl. 1977. *Selected Writings*. David McLellan, ed. Oxford: Oxford University Press.

Matthews, Ann M. 1987. "Widowhood as an Expectable Life Event." In Victor W. Marshall, ed. *Aging in Canada: Social Perspectives*, 343–66. Toronto: Fitzhenry and Whiteside.

Meeker, B. F. 1980. "Rational Decision-Making Models in Interpersonal Behavior." In T. K. Burch, ed. *Demographic Behavior: Interdisciplinary Perspectives on Decision-Making*. Boulder, CO: Westview.

Messinger, Hans, and Brian J. Powell. 1987. "The Implications of Canada's Aging Society on Social Expenditures." In Victor W. Marshall, ed. *Aging in Canada: Social Perspectives*, 569–85. Toronto: Fitzhenry and Whiteside.

Miller, J. Hillis. 1979. "The Critic as Host." In Harold Bloom et. al. *Deconstruction and Criticism*, 217–56. New York: Continuum.

Minkowsky, E. 1970. *Lived Time: Phenomenological and Psychopathological Studies.* Evanston: Northwestern University Press.

Minsky, M. 1981. "A Framework for Presenting Knowledge." In J. Haugeland, ed. *Mind Design.* Cambridge, MA: MIT Press.

Mizruchi, Ephraim H. 1983. "Abeyance Processes, Social Policy and Aging." In Anne-Marie Guillemard, ed., *Old Age and the Welfare State*, 45–52. Beverly Hills: Sage.

Monk, Abraham. 1980. "More on the Economics of Aging." In Edgar F. Borgatta and Neil G. McCluskey, eds. *Aging and Society*, 42–46. Beverly Hills: Sage.

Montgomery, Rhonda J. V. et. al. 1987. "Dependency, Family Extension, and Long-Term Care Policy." In Edgar F. Borgatta and Rhonda J. V. Montgomery, eds. *Critical Issues in Aging Policy*, 161–77. Beverly Hills: Sage.

Moran, Richard. 1989. "Seeing and Believing: Metaphor, Image, and Force." *Critical Inquiry* (16) Autumn:87–112.

Morgan, John C. 1979. *Becoming Old: An Introduction to Social Gerontology.* New York: Springer.

Morris, Charles W. 1946. *Signs, Language, and Behavior.* New York: Prentice-Hall.

Munnichs, Joep M. A. 1976. "Dependency, Interdependency and Autonomy: An Introduction." In J. Munnicks and Wim J. A. van den Heuvel, eds., *Dependency or Interdependency in Old Age*, 3–8. The Hague: Martinus Nijhoff, 1976.

Munnichs, Joep M. A., and Wim J. A. van den Heuvel, eds. 1976. *Dependency or Interdependency in Old Age.* The Hague: Martinus Nijhoff.

Myers, George C. 1985. "Aging and Worldwide Population Change." In Robert H. Binstock and E. Shanas, eds. *Handbook of Aging and the Social Sciences*, 173–198. New York: Van Nostrand Reinhold.

Myles, John. 1986. "Citizenship at the Crossroads: The Future of Old Age Security." In David van Tassel and Peter N. Stearns, eds. *Old Age in a Bureaucratic Society*, 193–216. CT: Greenwood.

Nascher, I. L. (1909). "Geriatrics." *New York Medical Journal* (90), Aug. 21:358–59.

Nelson, John S., Alan Magill, and Donald N. McClosky, eds. 1987. *The Rhetoric of the Human Sciences: Language and Argument in Scholarship and Public Affairs.* Madison: University of Wisconsin Press.

Nesdoly, Tracy. 1988. "The Greening of the Greys." *The Sunday Sun* (Toronto), Dec. 18: C9.

Neugarten, Bernice L. 1974. "Age Groups in American Society and the Rise of the Young-Old." *Annals of the American Academy of Political and Social Science* (415):187–98.

Neugarten, Bernice L. 1981. "Personality Change in Late Life: A Developmental Perspective." In C. Kart and B. Manard, eds. *Aging in America: Readings in Social Gerontology*, 208–32. 2nd ed., Sherman Oaks, CA: Alfred Sherman.

Neugarten, Bernice L. 1987. "Aging: Social Policy Issues for the Developed Countries." In Manfred Bergener et al., eds. *Aging into the Eighties and Beyond*, 391–401. New York: Springer.

Neugarten, Bernice L., Joan W. Moore, and John C. Lowe. 1965. "Age Norms,
    Age Constraints, and Adult Socialization." *American Journal of Sociology*
    (70):710–17.
Novak, Mark, 1988. *Aging and Society: A Canadian Perspective*. Toronto: Nelson.
Olson, Laura K. 1982. *The Political Economy of Aging*. New York: Columbia Uni-
    versity Press.
Ortony, Andrew, ed. 1979. *Metaphor and Thought*. Cambridge: Cambridge Uni-
    versity Press.
'Otiosus'. 1988. *The Idler* (Toronto), May/June:7.
Paillat, Paul. 1976. "Criteria of Independent (Autonomous) Life in Old Age." In
    J. Munnichs and W. van den Heuvel, eds. *Dependency or Interdependency in
    Old Age*, 35–41. The Hague: Martinus Nijhoff.
Paivio, Allan. 1979. "Psychological Processes in the Comprehension of Meta-
    phor." In A. Ortony, eds. *Metaphor and Thought*, 150–171. Cambridge: Cam-
    bridge University.
Palmore, Erdman, B. 1977. "Facts on Aging: A Short Quiz." *The Gerontologist*
    (19):169–74.
Parsons, Talcott. 1989. "A Tentative Outline of American Values." *Theory, Cul-
    ture, and Society* (6):577–612.
Pecheux, Michel. 1982. *Language, Semantics, and Ideology*. New York: St. Martin's.
Philibert, Michel. 1982. "The Phenomenological Approach to Images of Aging."
    In Patrick L. McKee, ed. *Philosophical Foundations of Aging*, 303–22. New
    York: Human Sciences Press.
Phillipson, Chris. 1982. *Capitalism and the Construction of Old Age*. London: Mac-
    millan.
Pike, Kenneth. 1954. *Language in Relation to a Unified Theory of the Structure of
    Human Action*. Glendale: University of California.
Pitkin, Hanna F. 1972. *Wittgenstein and Justice*. California: University of Califor-
    nia.
Polkinghorne, Donald E. 1988. *Narrative Knowing and the Human Sciences*. New
    York: SUNY Press.
Pollner, Melvin. 1987. *Mundane Reasoning: Reality in Everyday and Sociological
    Discourse*. Cambridge: Cambridge University Press.
Posner, Roland. 1982. *Rational Discourse and Poetic Communication*. New York:
    Mouton.
Pratt, Henry. 1976. *The Gray Lobby*. Chicago: University of Chicago Press.
Propp, Vladimir. 1968. *The Morphology of the Folk Tale*. Trans. by Lawrence Scott.
    Austin: University of Texas Press.
Prus, Robert. 1990. "The Interpretive Challenge: The Impending Crisis in Soci-
    ology." *Canadian Journal of Sociology* (15) Summer:355–63.
Putnam, Hilary. 1975. "The Meaning of 'Meaning'." In K. Gunderson, ed. *Min-
    nesota Studies in the Philosophy of Science*, Vol. 7, 135–151. Minneapolis: Uni-
    versity of Minnesota Press.
Quadagno, Jill. 1984. "Welfare Capitalism and the Social Security Act of 1935."
    American Sociological Review (49):632–47.
Quadagno, Jill. 1986. "The Transformation of Old Age Security." In D. van Tassel
    and P. N. Stearns, eds. *Old Age in a Bureaucratic Society*, 129–55. Norwalk
    CT: Greenwood.

Radbruch, Gestav. 1950. "Legal Philosophy." In *The Legal Philosophies of Lask, Radbruch, and Dabin*, 47–224. Trans. and edited by K. Wilks. Cambridge: Harvard University Press.

Rathbone-McCuan, Eloise, and Betty Havens, eds. 1988. *North American Elders: U.S. and Canadian Perspectives*. New York: Greenwood.

Reddy, Michael J. 1979. "The Conduit Metaphor—A Case of Frame Conflict in Our Language about Language." Pp. 284–324, in *Metaphor and Thought*, A. Ortony, ed. Cambridge: Cambridge University Press.

Reiss, Timothy. 1982. *The Discourse of Modernism*. Ithica: Cornell University Press.

Rickert, Heinrich. 1986. *The Limits of Concept Formation in Natural Science: A Logical Introduction to the Historical Sciences*. Trans. and ed. with an Introduction by Guy Oakes. New York: Cambridge University Press.

Ricoeur, Paul. 1971. "The Model of the Text: Meaningful Action Considered as a Text." *Social Research* (28):529–563.

Ricoeur, Paul. 1974. *The Conflict of Interpretations*. Evanston, IL: Northwestern University Press.

Ricoeur, Paul. 1976. *Interpretation Theory*. Fort Worth: Texas Christian University Press.

Ricoeur, Paul. 1977. *The Rule of Metaphor*. Toronto: University of Toronto Press.

Ricoeur, Paul. 1978. "Explanation and Understanding." In C. Reagan and D. Stewart, eds. *The Philosophy of Paul Ricoeur*, 158–186. Boston: Beacon.

Ricoeur, Paul, 1980. "Narrative Time." *Critical Inquiry* (7) Autumn:169–190.

Ricoeur, Paul. 1981. "The Narrative Function." In J. B. Thompson, ed. *Paul Ricoeur: Hermeneutics and the Human Sciences*, 274–96. New York: Cambridge University Press.

Ricoeur, Paul. 1986. "Habermas (2)." In George H. Taylor, ed. *Lectures on Ideology and Utopia*, New York: Columbia University Press.

Riffaterre, Michael. 1984. "Intertextual Representation: On Mimesis as Interpretive Discourse." *Critical Inquiry* (11) September:141–162.

Riffaterre, Michael. 1990. "Fear of Theory." *New Literary History* (21) Autumn:921–938.

Riley, Matilda White. 1985. "Age Strata in Social Systems." In R. H. Binstock and E. Shanas, eds. *Handbook of Aging and the Social Sciences*, 369–411. New York: Van Nostrand Reinhold.

Ritzer, George. 1988. *Contemporary Sociological Theory*, 2nd ed. New York: Alfred A. Knopf.

Rorty, Richard. 1980. *Philosophy and the Mirror of Nature*. Princeton: Princeton University Press.

Rose, Arnold. 1965. "The Subculture of the Aging: A Framework for Research in Social Gerontology." In A. Rose and W. Peterson, eds. *Older People and Their Social Worlds*, 3–16. Philadelphia: F. A. Davis.

Rosow, Irving. 1985. "Status and Role Change through the Life Cycle." In R. H. Binstock and E. Shanas, eds. *Handbook of Aging and the Social Sciences*, 62–93. New York: Van Nostrand Reinhold.

Ryff, Carol D. 1986. "The Subjective Construction of Self and Society: An Agenda for Life-Span Research." In Victor W. Marshall, ed. *Later Life: The Social Psychology of Aging*, 33–74. Beverly Hills, CA: Sage.

Sacks, Harvey. 1972a. "An Initial Investigation of the Usability of Conversational Data for Doing Sociology." In D. N. Sudnow, ed. *Studies in Social Interaction*, 31–74. New York: The Free Press.

Sacks, Harvey. 1984. "On Doing Being Ordinary." In J. M. Atkinson and J. C. Heritage, eds. *Structures of Social Action*, 413–529. Cambridge: Cambridge University Press.

Sacks, Harvey. 1989. "Lectures 1964–1965." Edited by Gail Jefferson with an Introduction/Memoir by E. A. Schegloff. *Human Studies* (12):3–4.

Saussure, Ferdinand de. 1959 [1916]. *Course in General Linguistics*. New York: Philosophical Library.

Schank, R. C., and R. P. Abelson. 1977. *Scripts, Plans, Goals, and Understanding*. Hillsdale, NJ: Lawrence Erlbaum.

Schleifer, Ronald. 1987. *A. J. Greimas and the Nature of Meaning*. Lincoln: University of Nebraska Press.

Scholes, Robert. 1977. "Towards a Semiotics of Literature." *Critical Inquiry* (4) Autumn:105–120.

Schön, Donald A. 1979. "Generative Metaphor: A Perspective on Problem-Setting in Social Policy." In A. Ortony, ed. *Metaphor and Thought*, 254–83. Cambridge: Cambridge University Press.

Schulz, Richard. 1989. Review of 'The Elderly as Modern Pioneers', edited by Philip Silverman. *Contemporary Sociology* (18) January:139–40.

Schütz, Alfred. 1967. *The Phenomenology of the Social World*. Evanston, IL: Northwestern University Press.

Schütz, Alfred. 1973. *Collected Papers I: The Problem of Social Reality*. The Hague: Martinus Nijhoff.

Searle, J. R. 1969. *Speech Acts*. Cambridge: Cambridge University Press.

Searle, J. R. 1979a. *Expression and Meaning*. Cambridge: Cambridge University Press.

Searle, J. R. 1979b. "Metaphor." In A. Ortony, ed., *Metaphor and Thought*, op. cit., 92–123. Cambridge: Cambridge University Press.

Shanas, Ethel. 1979. "The Family as a Social Support System in Old Age." *The Gerontologist* (19):169–174.

Shils, Edward. 1980. *The Calling of Sociology and Other Essays in the Pursuit of Learning*. Chicago: University of Chicago Press.

Simmel, Georg. 1971. *On Individuality and Social Forms*, D. Levine, ed. Chicago: University of Chicago Press.

Simmel, Georg. 1980. *Essays on Interpretation in Social Science*. Trans. by Guy Oakes. Totowa, NJ: Rowman and Littlefield.

Simon, Herbert. 1971. "Decision-Making and Organizational Design: Man-Machine Systems for Decision-Making." In D. S. Pugh, ed., *Organization Theory: Selected Readings*, 189–212. Baltimore: Penguin.

Simons, Herbert W. ed. 1989. *Rhetoric in the Human Sciences*. Newbury Park, CA: Sage.

Simons, Herbert W., ed. 1990. *The Rhetorical Turn: Invention and Persuasion in the Conduct of Inquiry*. Chicago: University of Chicago Press.

Simons, Ronald C., and Charles C. Hughes, eds. 1985. *The Culture-Bound Syndromes*. Boston: D. Reidel.

Smith, Dorothy E. 1990a. *The Conceptual Practices of Power: A Feminist Sociology of Knowledge*. Boston: Northeastern University Press.

Smith, Dorothy E. 1990b. *Texts, Facts, and Femininity: Exploring the Relations of Ruling*. New York: Routledge.

Solem, Erik. 1976. "Dependency—Due to Lack of Individual or Environmental Resources." In, J. Munnichs and J. van den Heuvel, eds., *Dependency or Interdependency in Old Age*, 71–79. The Hague: Martinus Nijhoff.

Specht, Ernst K. 1969. *The Foundations of Wittgenstein's Late Philosophy*. Manchester: Manchester University Press.

Spence, Donald L. 1986. "Some Contributions of Symbolic Interaction to the Study of Growing Old." In Victor W. Marshall, ed. *Later Life: The Social Psychology of Aging*, 107–124. Beverly Hills, CA: Sage.

Sprinker, Michael. 1980. "The Use and Abuse of Foucault." *Humanities in Society* (3) Winter:1–22.

Stern, Laurent. 1990. "Narrative versus Description in Historiography." *New Literary History* (21) Spring:555–568.

Stone, Leroy O., and Susan Fletcher. 1987. "The Hypothesis of Age Patterns in Living Arrangement Passages." In Victor W. Marshall, ed. *Aging in Canada: Social Perspectives*, 288–310. Toronto: Fitzhenry and Whiteside.

Strehler, B. 1977. *Time, Cells and Aging*, 2nd. ed. New York: Academic Press.

Streib, Gordon F. 1965. "Are the Aged a Minority Group?" In Alvin W. Gouldner and S. M. Miller, eds. *Applied Sociology*, 311–28. New York: Free Press.

Streib, Gordon F. 1985. "Social Stratification and Aging." In R. H. Binstock and E. Shanas, eds. *Handbook of Aging and the Social Sciences*, 339–68. New York: Van Nostrand Reinhold.

Streib, Gordon F., and Harold L. Orbach. 1967. "Aging." In Paul F. Lazarsfeld, William H. Sewell, and Harold L. Wilensky, eds. *The Uses of Sociology* 612–640. New York: Basic Books.

Sunday Telegraph. 1988. "Paradise—or Purgatory?" April 24:22.

Szemberg, Alexander. 1988. "The Stainless Swedes." *The Idler*, September/October:10–17.

Taylor, Charles. 1985. *Human Agency and Language*. Cambridge, MA: Cambridge University Press.

Thomas, Eugene L., Patricia A. Kraus, and Kim O. Chambers. 1990. "Metaphoric Analysis of Meaning in the Lives of Elderly Men: A Cross-Cultural Investigation." *Journal of Aging Studies* (4):1–15.

Toronto Life. 1988. "Growing Old Gracefully." May:52–55, 81–85.

Toronto Sun. 1987. "They're Super Seniors." Monday, Oct. 26:43.

Treas, Judith, 1981. "Family Support Systems for the Aged: Some Social and Demographic Considerations." In C. Kart and B. Manard, eds. *Aging in America*, 327–37. Sherman Oaks, CA: Alfred Sherman.

Tropman, John E. 1987. *Public Policy Opinion and the Elderly, 1952–1978: A Kaleidescope of Culture*. New York: Greenwood Press.

Turner, Victor W. 1980. "Social Dramas and Stories about Them." *Critical Inquiry* (7) Autumn:141–68.

Turner, Victor W., and Edward M. Bruner, eds. 1986. *The Anthropology of Experience*. Urbana, IL: University of Illinois Press.

Ujimoto, Victor K. 1987. "The Ethnic Dimension of Aging in Canada." In Victor W. Marshall, *Aging in Canada: Social Perspectives*, 2nd ed. Toronto: Fitzhenry and Whiteside.

van den Heuvel, Wim J. A. 1976. "The Meaning of Dependency." In J. Munnichs and W. van den Heuvel, eds. *Dependency or Interdependency in Old Age*, 162–73. The Hague: Martinus Nijhoff.

van Dijk, Teun A. 1972. *Some Aspects of Text Grammars*. The Hague: Mouton.

van Dijk, Teun A. 1977. *Text and Context*. London: Longman.

van Dijk, Teun A., and Walter Kintsch. 1983. *Strategies of Discourse Comprehension*. New York: Academic Press.

van Tassel, David, and Peter N. Stearns, eds. 1986. *Old Age in a Bureaucratic Society*. New York: Greenwood Press.

Walker, Allan. 1983. "Social Policy and Elderly People in Great Britain: The Construction of Dependent Social and Economic Status in Old Age." In Anne-Marie Guillemard, ed. *Old Age and the Welfare State*, 143–68. Beverly Hills: Sage.

Weber, Max. 1978. *Economy and Society*, 2 vols. G. Roth and C. Wittich, eds. Berkeley: University of California Press.

Weimann, Robert. 1988. "Text, Author-Function, and Appropriation in Modern Narrative: Toward a Sociology of Representation." *Critical Inquiry* (14) Spring:431–147.

Wershow, Harold J., ed. 1981. *Controversial Issues in Gerontology*. New York: Springer.

White, Hayden. 1978. *Tropics of Discourse*. Baltimore: Johns Hopkins.

White, Hayden. 1980. "The Value of Narrativity in the Representation of Reality." *Critical Inquiry* (7) Autumn:5–28.

Whorf, Benjamin Lee. 1956. *Language, Thought and Reality*, J. Carroll, ed. Cambridge, MA: M.I.T. Press.

Wieder, D. Lawrence. 1974. *Language and Reality*. The Hague: Mouton.

Wilkins, Russell, and Owen Adams. 1983. "Health Expectancy in Canada, Late 1970's: Demographic, Regional and Social Dimensions." *American Journal of Public Health* (73): 1073–1080.

Wister, Andrew V., and Thomas K. Burch. 1987. "Values, Perceptions, and Choice in Living Arrangements of the Elderly." In E. Borgatta and R. Montgomery, eds. *Critical Issues in Aging Policy*, 178–98. Beverly Hills: Sage.

Wittgenstein, Ludwig. 1976. *Philosophical Investigations*, 2nd ed. Oxford: Basil Blackwell.

Woolgar, Steve, ed. 1988. *Knowledge and Reflexivity: New Frontiers in the Sociology of Knowledge*. London: Sage.

Wyatt-Brown, Anne M. 1989. "The Narrative Imperative: Fiction and the Aging Writer." *Journal of Aging Studies* (3):55–65.

Index